Milton L. Wainberg, MD
Andrew J. Kolodny, MD
Jack Drescher, MD
Editors

Crystal Meth and Men Who Have Sex with Men: What Mental Health Care Professionals Need to Know

Crystal Meth and Men Who Have Sex with Men: What Mental Health Care Professionals Need to Know has been co-published simultaneously as *Journal of Gay & Lesbian Psychotherapy*, Volume 10, Numbers 3/4 2006.

Pre-publication REVIEWS, COMMENTARIES, EVALUATIONS . . .

More pre-publication
REVIEWS, COMMENTARIES, EVALUATIONS . . .

"A NECESSARY READ FOR ALL MEDICAL AND MENTAL HEALTH PRACTITIONERS working to reduce the spread of HIV and to care for men who have sex with men. . . . IT IS UNIQUE IN ITS MIX OF PROFESSIONAL, MEDICAL IN-FORMATION WITH THE PERSONAL ACCOUNTS of those whose lives have been profoundly affected by the most dangerous drug of abuse to spread in modern times. . . . POWER-FUL FIRST PERSON NARRATIVES il-lustrate the damage done to people who struggle with crystal meth ad-diction every day. The deepest psy-chological themes of isolation, despair, loneliness, and self loathing confront the reader's attempt to make sense out of an epidemic of substance abuse that threatens to undo any gains we have made in the epidemic. The power of such personal accounts precludes the complete intellectual-ization of the epidemic, forcing us to confront the most difficult questions about addiction, self care, and group psychology. In addition to providing an enormous amount of useful clini-cal information, this volume will force all mental health clinicians to think more deeply about the complexity of crystal meth's impact on the body, brain, mind and spirit."

Marshall Forstein, MD
Associate Professor of Psychiatry
Harvard Medical School
Director
Adult Psychiatry Residency Training
The Cambridge Hospital,
The Cambridge Health Alliance

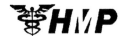

The Haworth Medical Press®
An Imprint of The Haworth Press, Inc.

Crystal Meth and Men Who Have Sex with Men: What Mental Health Care Professionals Need to Know

Crystal Meth and Men Who Have Sex with Men: What Mental Health Care Professionals Need to Know has been co-published simultaneously as *Journal of Gay & Lesbian Psychotherapy*, Volume 10, Numbers 3/4 2006.

1. *Addictions in the Gay and Lesbian Community*, edited by Jeffrey R. Guss, MD, and Jack Drescher, MD (Vol. 3, No. 3/4, 2000). *Explores the unique clinical considerations involved in addiction treatment for gay men and lesbians, groups that reportedly use and abuse alcohol and substances at higher rates than the general population.*

2. *Gay and Lesbian Parenting*, edited by Deborah F. Glazer, PhD, and Jack Drescher, MD (Vol. 4, No. 3/4, 2001). *Richly textured, probing. These papers accomplish a rare feat: they explore in a candid, psychologically sophisticated, yet highly readable fashion how parenthood impacts lesbian and gay identity and how these identities affect the experience of parenting. Wonderfully informative. (Martin Stephen Frommer, PhD, Faculty/Supervisor, The Institute for Contemporary Psychotherapy, New York City).*

3. *Sexual Conversion Therapy: Ethical, Clinical, and Research Perspectives*, edited by Ariel Shidlo, PhD, Michael Schroeder, PsyD, and Jack Drescher, MD (Vol. 5, No. 3/4, 2001). *"This is an important book. . . . an invaluable resource for mental health providers and policymakers. This book gives voice to those men and women who have experienced painful, degrading, and unsuccessful conversion therapy and survived. The ethics and misuses of conversion therapy practice are well documented, as are the harmful effects." (Joyce Hunter, DSW, Research Scientist, HIV Center for Clinical & Behavioral Studies, New York State Psychiatric Institute/ Columbia University, New York City)*

4. *The Mental Health Professions and Homosexuality: International Perspectives*, edited by Vittorio Lingiardi, MD, and Jack Drescher, MD (Vol. 7, No. 1/2, 2003). *"Provides a worldwide perspective that illuminates the psychiatric, psychoanalytic, and mental health professions' understanding and treatment of both lay and professional sexual minorities." (Bob Barrett, PhD, Professor and Counseling Program Coordinator, University of North Carolina at Charlotte)*

5. *Transgender Subjectivities: A Clinician's Guide*, edited by Ubaldo Leli, MD, and Jack Drescher, MD (Vol. 8, No. 1/2, 2004). *"Indispensable for diagnosticians and therapists dealing with gender dysphoria, important for researchers, and a direct source of help for all individuals suffering from painful uncertainties regarding their sexual identity." (Otto F. Kernberg, MD, Director, Personality Disorders Institute, Weill Medical College of Cornell University)*

6. *Handbook of LGBT Issues in Community Mental Health*, edited by Ronald E. Hellman, MD, and Jack Drescher, MD (Vol. 8, No. 3/4, 2004). *"Comprehensive . . . Richly strewn with data, useful addresses of voluntary and other organizations, and case histories." (Michael King, MD, PhD, Professor of Primary Care Psychiatry, Royal Free and University College Medical School, London)*

7. *A Gay Man's Guide to Prostate Cancer*, edited by Gerald Perlman, PhD, and Jack Drescher, MD (Vol. 9, No. 1/2, 2005). *"Excellent. . . . highly recommended. Patients reading this book will find themselves here, and professionals will learn what they need to help their patients as they struggle with these emotional topics." (Donald Johannessen, MD, Clinical Assistant Professor of Psychiatry, NYU School of Medicine)*

8. *Barebacking: Psychosocial and Public Health Approaches*, edited by Perry N. Halkitis, PhD, Leo Wilton, PhD, and Jack Drescher, MD (Vol. 9, No. 3/4, 2005). *An examination of the psychological, social, and health issues involving intentional unprotected gay or bisexual sex.*

9. *Crystal Meth and Men Who Have Sex with Men: What Mental Health Care Professionals Need to Know,* edited by Milton L. Wainberg, MD, Andrew J. Kolodny, MD, and Jack Drescher, MD (Vol. 10, No. 3/4, 2006). *"This comprehensive book captures not just the extent of the problem and how to recognize it, it offers excellent clinical interventions and treatments. . . . invaluable." (Robert Paul Cabaj, MD, Director, San Francisco Department of Public Health's Community Behavioral Health Services, Member, Mayor's Task Force on Methamphetamine Abuse, San Francisco)*

Crystal Meth and Men Who Have Sex with Men: What Mental Health Care Professionals Need to Know

Milton L. Wainberg, MD
Andrew J. Kolodny, MD
Jack Drescher, MD
Editors

Crystal Meth and Men Who Have Sex with Men: What Mental Health Care Professionals Need to Know has been co-published simultaneously as *Journal of Gay & Lesbian Psychotherapy*, Volume 10, Numbers 3/4 2006.

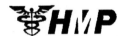

The Haworth Medical Press®
Harrington Park Press®
Imprints of The Haworth Press, Inc.

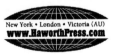

New York • London • Victoria (AU)
www.HaworthPress.com

Published by

The Haworth Medical Press®, 10 Alice Street, Binghamton, NY 13904-1580 USA

The Haworth Medical Press® is an imprint of The Haworth Press, Inc., 10 Alice Street, Binghamton, NY 13904-1580 USA.

Crystal Meth and Men Who Have Sex with Men: What Mental Health Care Professionals Need to Know has been co-published simultaneously as *Journal of Gay & Lesbian Psychotherapy*, Volume 10, Numbers 3/4 2006.

Cover design by Jennifer Gaska.

Library of Congress Cataloging-in-Publication Data

Crystal meth and men who have sex with men : what mental health care professionals need to know / Milton L. Wainberg, Andrew J. Kolodny, Jack Drescher, editors.
     p. cm.
     "Co-published simultaneously as Journal of gay & lesbian psychotherapy, volume10, numbers 3/4, 2006."
     Includes bibliographical references and index.
     ISBN-13: 978-0-7890-3247-8 (hard cover : alk. paper)
     ISBN-10: 0-7890-3247-3 (hard cover : alk. paper)
     ISBN-13: 978-0-7890-3248-5 (soft cover : alk. paper)
     ISBN-10: 0-7890-3248-1 (soft cover : alk. paper)
     1. Gay men–Substance use–United States. 2. Gay men–Drug use–United States. 3. Gay men–Sexual behavior–United States. 4. Methamphetamine abuse–United States. 5. AIDS (Disease)–Risk factors–United States. 6. Safe sex in AIDS prevention–United States. I. Wainberg, Milton L. II. Kolodny, Andrew J. III. Drescher, Jack, 1951- IV. Journal of gay & lesbian psychotherapy.
RC564.5.G39C79 2006
362.29'9–dc22

                                    2005032411

Indexing, Abstracting & Website/Internet Coverage

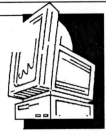

This section provides you with a list of major indexing & abstracting services and other tools for bibliographic access. That is to say, each service began covering this periodical during the year noted in the right column. Most Websites which are listed below have indicated that they will either post, disseminate, compile, archive, cite or alert their own Website users with research-based content from this work. (This list is as current as the copyright date of this publication.)

(continued)

(continued)

*Special Bibliographic Notes related to special journal issues
(separates) and indexing/abstracting:*

- indexing/abstracting services in this list will also cover material in any "separate" that is co-published simultaneously with Haworth's special thematic journal issue or DocuSerial. Indexing/abstracting usually covers material at the article/chapter level.
- monographic co-editions are intended for either non-subscribers or libraries which intend to purchase a second copy for their circulating collections.
- monographic co-editions are reported to all jobbers/wholesalers/approval plans. The source journal is listed as the "series" to assist the prevention of duplicate purchasing in the same manner utilized for books-in-series.
- to facilitate user/access services all indexing/abstracting services are encouraged to utilize the co-indexing entry note indicated at the bottom of the first page of each article/chapter/contribution.
- this is intended to assist a library user of any reference tool (whether print, electronic, online, or CD-ROM) to locate the monographic version if the library has purchased this version but not a subscription to the source journal.
- individual articles/chapters in any Haworth publication are also available through the Haworth Document Delivery Service (HDDS).

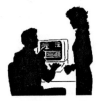

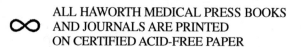

Crystal Meth and Men Who Have Sex with Men: What Mental Health Care Professionals Need to Know

CONTENTS

ABOUT THE EDITORS

Milton L. Wainberg, MD, is Associate Clinical Professor of Psychiatry at the Columbia College of Physicians and Surgeons. He is the Medical Director of the Columbia University HIV Mental Health Training Project; in that capacity, he has trained several hundred medical, HIV, and mental health care providers about clinical issues at the intersection of HIV and mental health, and has done research to identify gaps in HIV-related service provision in mental health care agencies. He is a member of the American Psychiatric Association Committee on AIDS and Vice-Chair of the Mental Health HIV Clinical Guidelines Committee NYS Department of Health AIDS Institute.

Dr. Wainberg has expertise in international research developing HIV prevention interventions psychiatric patients in South Africa and Brazil; for the latter, he is the Principal Investigator of an NIMH-funded R01: "Brazilian HIV Prevention for the Severely Mentally Ill." He also has experience in several NIAA, NIDA and CDC funded HIV prevention research with gay and bisexual men who are using alcohol, recreational drugs or have sexual compulsivity.

Andrew J. Kolodny, MD, is the Vice Chairman for Clinical Psychiatry in the Department of Psychiatry at the Maimonides Medical Center. He was the Medical Director for Special Projects in the Office of the Executive Deputy Commissioner at the NYC Department of Health and Mental Hygiene (DOHMH). Dr. Kolodny leads the Department's Buprenorphine Initiative, as well as other special projects to reduce morbidity and mortality from substance and alcohol use. He Chairs the Public Psychiatry Committee of the NY County District Branch of the American Psychiatric Association. Dr. Kolodny was a Congressional Health Policy Fellow in the United States Senate. He has a clinical practice specializing in the treatment of substance use disorders.

Jack Drescher, MD, is a Fellow, Training, and Supervising Analyst at the William Alanson White Psychoanalytic Institute. He is Adjunct Clinical Assistant Professor at New York University Postdoctoral Program in Psychotherapy and Psychoanalysis. He is Past President of the

New York County District Branch, American Psychiatric Association and Past Chair of the Committee on GLB Concerns of the APA. Dr. Drescher is a Distinguished Fellow of the APA. Author of *Psychoanalytic Therapy and the Gay Man* (1998, The Analytic Press), and Editor-in-Chief of the *Journal of Gay & Lesbian Psychotherapy*. Dr. Drescher is in private practice in New York City.

Introduction:
A Look Inside the "Crystal" Ball

This special publication of the *Journal of Gay & Lesbian Psychotherapy* takes a hard look at the abuse of methamphetamine (MA), popularly known as "crystal," "crystal meth," or "Tina." As we write these words, there has been much in the news recently on the subject of methamphetamine–and for good reason. Some have declared MA the nation's leading law enforcement scourge; it is blamed for crowding jails, fueling increases in theft and violence and other social problems (New York Times, 2005).

In recent years, there has been an increase in methamphetamine use among men who have sex with men (MSM) and the data shows that where there is MA use, increases in sexual risk behaviors for HIV and other sexually transmitted infections (STIs) often follow. The *JGLP* recently devoted a special issue to the subject of barebacking (unprotected anal intercourse or UAI) among gay men (Volume 9, Numbers 3/4, 2005; also available as Halkitis, Wilton and Drescher, 2005). There, MA was frequently cited as a contributing factor in increased sexual risk-taking. Both MA users and the clinicians who treat them note that the drug has appealing, powerful qualities–including a potent sense of connection, increases in general energy level, libido surge and sexual energy that last for hours. All of these factors make MA an addictive drug which is very difficult to stop using. When these qualities are combined with unsafe sexual activity, the drug then acquires a prominent role in STI and HIV

[Haworth co-indexing entry note]: "Introduction: A Look Inside the 'Crystal' Ball." Wainberg, Milton L., Andrew J. Kolodny, and Jack Drescher. Co-published simultaneously in *Journal of Gay & Lesbian Psychotherapy* (The Haworth Medical Press, an imprint of The Haworth Press, Inc.) Vol. 10, No. 3/4, 2006, pp. 1-7; and: *Crystal Meth and Men Who Have Sex with Men: What Mental Health Care Professionals Need to Know* (ed: Milton L. Wainberg, Andrew J. Kolodny, and Jack Drescher) The Haworth Medical Press, an imprint of The Haworth Press, Inc., 2006, pp. 1-7. Single or multiple copies of this article are available for a fee from The Haworth Document Delivery Service [1-800-HAWORTH, 9:00 a.m. - 5:00 p.m. (EST). E-mail address: docdelivery@haworthpress.com].

doi:10.1300/J236v10n03_01

transmission. In fact, after years of declining rates of new HIV infections among MSM, MA use may be fueling a resurgence in the AIDS epidemic among their number (Centers for Disease Control, 2005; Catania et al., 2001). On February 11, 2005, The New York City Department of Health and Mental Hygiene called attention to the association between MA use and HIV in announcing a case of resistant rapidly progressive HIV in a gay man who reported multiple male sex partners and unprotected anal intercourse while using methamphetamine (*http://www.nyc.gov/html/ doh/html/pr/pr016-05.shtml*).

This monograph of the *Journal of Gay & Lesbian Psychotherapy* aims to address and shed some light upon important issues surrounding MA use in the MSM community and the need to promptly act at a personal, individual and community level.[1] Methamphetamine poses a unique threat to the health of the MSM community because its use often leads rapidly to the downward spiral of addiction and because of its strong association with high-risk sexual behaviors. HIV prevention strategies employed by health departments in New York City and on the West Coast now include efforts to prevent MSM from ever starting to use MA and efforts to ensure that methamphetamine-addicted MSM have prompt access to gay-affirmative substance abuse treatment programs. As many of the contributors to this volume attest, ample evidence exists that substance abuse treatment programs offering methamphetamine-addicted MSM an opportunity to openly and safely discuss sexual behaviors associated with their drug use can effectively reduce high-risk sexual behaviors and promote safer sexual practices.

This monograph is aimed not only at the mental health professionals who may treat MSM, it is also intended to educate patients, their partners and relatives, as well as other medical and health care specialists who treat them. This volume contains the published proceedings of two important community events that took place in New York City in the year 2004. The first is *The Crystal Meth-HIV Connection: A Public Forum with Harvey Fierstein* (http://www.hivforumnyc.org/hivconnection.php). This public forum, organized by Dan Carlson and Bruce Kellerhouse, addressed the most prevalent concern voiced by those in attendance at a previous Forum held November 16, 2003 (i.e., methamphetamine binges are fueling the rise of new HIV infections). There were 700 people in attendance at the forum, including concerned individuals and representatives from city and government, and gay community service organizations.

Harvey Fierstein, the award-winning actor, writer, producer, and activist whose Broadway credits include *Torch Song Trilogy, La Cage Aux Folles, Hairspray*, and *Fiddler on the Roof*, moderated the forum. Forum panelists included Peter Staley, AIDS Activist and founder of AIDSMeds. com; Trevor P., a community member in recovery, Steven Lee, MD, a psychiatrist and addiction specialist, and Dr. Steven Tierney, Director of HIV Prevention for the San Francisco Department of Health. After the panelists' remarks, a town-hall meeting followed that included a range of audience responses from mental health workers, public health workers, government officials, individuals recovering from MA addiction, and concerned citizens. One reason for publishing the forum in this monograph is that it provides a model for community action for those communities that have not yet begun to address this issue. For example, the forum successfully highlighted the need to better inform the New York City MSM community about the dangers of MA use and the need to overcome barriers to changing behaviors and social norms. Following the event, forum organizers and other community-based organizations began collaborating closely with the New York City Department of Health and Mental Hygiene on the development and implementation of MA prevention campaigns.

The remaining papers in this publication were originally presented at another public meeting, *Crystal Methamphetamine: Understanding and Treating an Emerging Health Crisis.* This conference was sponsored by the NYC Department of Health and Mental Hygiene, the Centers for Diseases Control and Prevention and the Region II STD/HIV Prevention Training Center and took place on June 16, 2004.

We begin with "Crystal Meth Testimony" by Peter Staley, a personal account of his MA addiction from the perspective of a gay man who is also an AIDS community activist. Staley describes his first encounter with MA, the consequences of using it, treatment strategies he found helpful, and offers clinicians a patient's perspective on what they can do to prevent and treat MA use.

Following these personal and community accounts, the second section of this monograph includes presentations specifically dealing with the medical and psychiatric issues related to crystal use, abuse and dependence. This section begins with Antonio Urbina, MD's "Medical Complications of Crystal Methamphetamine." This paper reviews the available literature on the medical morbidity and mortality associated with MA abuse in HIV-infected patients–including hypertension, hyperthermia, rhabdomyolysis, stroke, and even death.

In "Methamphetamine Emergencies," Paul L. DeSandre, DO, details the alarming rise in emergency department visits related to MA use and notes that the problem is escalating in New York City in particular. He notes that patients may present to emergency departments in psychotic states, with seizures, strokes, or heart attacks. They may be in respiratory distress or in kidney failure. The toxic effects of the drug can be fatal. He notes that early recognition and basic interventions can be life sustaining, so it is important for clinicians to understand the range of toxicity and basic management strategies. As patients requiring emergency care are often in crisis and may be more receptive to intervention, he suggests that when discharging a patient from the emergency department, a "brief intervention" strategy may be effective at establishing that a problem exists, preventing future risk, and beginning recovery.

Next is "Psychiatric Consequences of Methamphetamine Use" by Andrew J. Kolodny, MD. This paper describes the adverse psychiatric consequences of MA abuse and the frequent co-occurring psychiatric disorders in those who present for mental health treatment. Although effective pharmacological treatments for methamphetamine dependence are not yet available, addressing the co-occurring psychiatric disorders (e.g., anxiety and mood disorders) improves MA treatment outcomes.

Susan Blank, MD, MPH, is the author of the final paper in this section with "Crystal Methamphetamine Use and Sexually Transmitted Infection: The Importance of Sexual History Taking." She argues that history-taking and screening for STIs can be a powerful way for primary care clinicians to identify and address MA and other substance abuse problems. As the majority of STIs have no noticeable symptoms in their early stages, clinicians diagnosing methamphetamine or other substance abuse problems, or taking care of the primary care needs of such patients should be familiar with sexual history-taking in order to identify patients needing a thorough exam and to ensure adequate STI screening.

The next section addresses crystal use prevalence and HIV seroconversion with which it is associated. As noted above, rates of high-risk sexual behavior are increasing since the late 1990s. In "Crystal Methamphetamine Use Among Men Who Have Sex with Men: Results from Two National Online Studies," Sabina Hirshfield, PhD, Robert H. Remien, PhD and Mary Ann Chiasson, DrPH, report on two web-based surveys of MSM recruited online. They found MA use was more likely to be associated with young age, having a greater number of sex partners, having unprotected anal intercourse (UAI), having a sexually transmitted infection (STI), and being HIV-positive.

In "Methamphetamine Use, Sexual Behavior, and HIV Seroconversion," Perry N. Halkitis, PhD, Kelly A. Green, MPH, and Daniel J. Carragher, PhD, as part of a larger, longitudinal study of club drug use among gay and bisexual men in New York City, assessed the sexual risk taking of those who identified as methamphetamine users. A subset of these men, who reported either a seronegative or unknown HIV status, was confirmed to be HIV-positive. Comparisons of this group to confirmed HIV-negative MA-using men in this study's sample indicated that these not known to be HIV-positive individuals differed in their reasons for MA use and in terms of their sexual risk taking. In particular, those who had seroconverted reported higher levels of unprotected receptive anal intercourse while high. Their study supports the belief that MA may play a causal role in HIV infection and may fuel the HIV epidemic at large.

The last section of this monograph focuses on ongoing efforts to find effective interventions and treatment strategies and models intended to reduce MA use and sexual risk behaviors. In "Club Drug Use and Risky Sex Among Gay and Bisexual Men in New York City," José E. Nanín, EdD, and Jeffrey T. Parsons, PhD, describe several studies conducted at the Center for HIV Educational Studies and Training (CHEST) at Hunter College of City University of New York that address prevalence of club drug use and unsafe sexual behaviors among various samples of gay and bisexual men in New York City. They make the case that creative educational interventions as well as clinical strategies using Motivational Interviewing and Cognitive Behavioral Therapy may be useful for clinicians and other health care practitioners by helping clients develop skills to reduce club drug use and risky sex.

Sherry Larkins, PhD, Cathy J. Reback, PhD, and Steven Shoptaw, PhD are next with "HIV Risk Behaviors Among Gay Male Methamphetamine Users: Before and After Treatment." They report on substance abuse treatment interventions that target both substance use and sexual behavior that have been successful in helping gay men reduce their sexual risks. They argue that such approaches have the potential to curtail the spread of HIV and other STIs, while simultaneously treating the substance abuse disorder.

Thomas W. Irwin, PhD, in "Strategies for the Treatment of Methamphetamine Use Disorders Among Gay and Bisexual Men," describes the significant barriers for MA users to engage in treatment and comments on several models of treatment that have been shown some success. These include motivational interviewing (MI), cognitive behavioral therapy (CBT), and community reinforcement with contingency management. Similarly, Donald A. Bux Jr., PhD and Thomas W. Irwin, PhD's "Combining Motivational Interviewing and Cognitive-Behavioral Skills Training for the Treatment of Crystal Methamphetamine Abuse/Dependence" presents the rationale and basic strategies encompassed by both MI and skills-based treatment approaches.

Jean Malpas, MA and Barbara E. Warren, PsyD, bring the voice of a gay community service organization to the discussion. Their paper, "Understanding and Treating the Crystal Methamphetamine Emerging Health Crisis: Using Community-Based Resources at the Lesbian, Gay, Bisexual and Transgender Community Center" shows how gay-identified community-based programs can provide a viable resource within which to develop and deliver the services needed to address the MA gay community problem. In an era of shrinking budgets, they emphasize the need for more resources and funding to meet the growing demand.

Finally, L. Donald McVinney, MSSW, MPhil, in "Harm Reduction, Crystal Methamphetamine, and Gay Men" writes on the changing definitions and models of harm reduction along with their practice applications providing an overview of harm reduction strategies for methamphetamine-using gay men.

Scientists, clinicians and community leaders–all represented in this monograph–report that crystal meth use makes HIV and other STI prevention efforts difficult to accomplish. Effective new medical treatments have produced significant declines in progression from HIV infection to AIDS (i.e., AIDS incidence) and in AIDS deaths, but these declines are slowing, indicating that much of the benefit of new therapies has been realized. Because HIV is transmitted through sexual and drug-use behaviors that encompass issues of human identity, pleasure, and need, making changes to prevent exposure to HIV can be difficult to initiate and sustain. Methamphetamine's impact on sexual behavior and its strong addiction potential pose a challenge to the task of improving the health of the gay community. Our goals in editing this special monograph publication of the *Journal of Gay & Lesbian Psychotherapy* are to raise awareness, to increase knowledge, to encourage further research and to stimulate ongoing participation in helping to improve the health status of our community.

Milton L. Wainberg, MD
Andrew J. Kolodny, MD
Jack Drescher, MD

NOTE

1. Very little has been documented about crystal use among lesbians and the possible specific adverse consequences the drug may have on the lesbian community. Some of the addictive and medical issues are probably the same (neither female gender nor lesbian specific adverse consequences have been published) and the potential STI/HIV transmission issues of lesbians may be exacerbated with crystal use.

REFERENCES

Catania J.A., Osmond D., Stall R.D., Pollack, L., Paul, J.P., Blower, S., Binson, D., Canchola, J.A., Mills, T.C., Fisher, L., Choi, K.H., Porco, T., Turner, C., Blair, J., Henne, J.L., Bye, L.L. & Coates, T.J. (2001), The continuing HIV epidemic among men who have sex with men. *American J. Public Health*, 91(6):907-914.

Centers for Disease Control and Prevention (2004), *Cases of HIV Infection and AIDS in the United States: 2003 HIV/AIDS Surveillance Report, Vol. 15*. Atlanta: US Department of Health and Human Services.

New York Times (2005), National Report. *New York Times*, July 6, p. A12.

Halkits, P.N., Wilton, L. & Drescher, J. (2005), *Barebacking: Psychosocial and Public Health Approaches*. New York: The Haworth Press, Inc.

A Public Forum–
Challenging the Culture of Disease:
The Crystal Meth-HIV Connection

Harvey Fierstein
Dan Carlson
Bruce Kellerhouse, PhD
Peter Staley
Trevor P.
Steven Tierney, EdD
Steven Lee, MD

Harvey Fierstein is an award-winning actor, writer, producer, and activist whose stage credits include *Torch Song Trilogy, La Cage Aux Folles, Hairspray,* and *Fiddler on the Roof.* Most recently he received the 2003 Drama Desk Award for Best Actor in a Musical, Drama League Award, and Tony Award for Best Actor in a Musical, making him the second person in history to win Tony's in four different categories.

Dan Carlson is Co-Founder of HIV Forum, and a member of the Crystal Meth Working Group.

Bruce Kellerhouse, a psychologist, is Co-Founder of HIV Forum and a member of the Crystal Meth Working Group.

Peter Staley created and paid for the ad campaign, *Huge Sale, Buy Crystal, Get HIV Free.* His website, AIDSmeds.com, offers treatment information for people living with HIV.

Trevor P. is a member of the gay recovery community.

Steven Tierney is Director of HIV Prevention for the City of San Francisco and Co-Chair of the State of California HIV Prevention Planning Group.

Steven Lee is Assistant Clinical Professor of Psychiatry, Columbia University and a Fellow of the American Academy of Addiction Psychiatrists.

This public forum was held on February 8, 2004 at the Haft Auditorium of the Fashion Institute of Technology (FIT) in New York City.

[Haworth co-indexing entry note]: "A Public Forum–Challenging the Culture of Disease: The Crystal Meth-HIV Connection." Fierstein, Harvey et al. Co-published simultaneously in *Journal of Gay & Lesbian Psychotherapy* (The Haworth Medical Press, an imprint of The Haworth Press, Inc.) Vol. 10, No. 3/4, 2006, pp. 9-43; and: *Crystal Meth and Men Who Have Sex with Men: What Mental Health Care Professionals Need to Know* (ed: Milton L. Wainberg, Andrew J. Kolodny, and Jack Drescher) The Haworth Medical Press, an imprint of The Haworth Press, Inc., 2006, pp. 9-43. Single or multiple copies of this article are available for a fee from The Haworth Document Delivery Service [1-800-HAWORTH, 9:00 a.m. - 5:00 p.m. (EST). E-mail address: docdelivery@haworthpress.com].

SUMMARY. Following a 2003 community forum on unsafe sexual practices among gay men, a follow up community forum was held on February 8, 2004 to address the insufficiently studied linkage between unsafe sexual practices, HIV transmission and crystal methamphetamine abuse. The forum was moderated by award-winning playwright and actor, Harvey Fierstein. The forum begins with an introduction by one of the organizers, Dan Carlson, who describes the forum as designed for private citizens to come together, identify with each other and talk about their experiences with crystal methamphetamine and to begin the process of formulating solutions to its widespread abuse. The other conference organizer, Bruce Kellerhouse, PhD, addressed the issue of inadequate public health messages to fight the increased use of crystal meth and an associated rise in HIV infections. He is followed by Peter Staley, an AIDS activist who used his own funds to finance a highly-visible advertising campaign warning of the linkage between crystal meth and HIV. "Trevor P." then recounts his personal experience as a gay man who HIV seroconverted while using crystal meth and who is now in recovery. Steven Tierney, EdD, next discusses obstacles in public health efforts to curb the spread of substance abuse and HIV infection. He also describes public health campaigns used in San Francisco. Steven Lee, MD, discusses psychiatric, psychological and pharmacological issues related to crystal methamphetamine addiction and HIV. The forum then is opened up to the general community, prompting a range of responses from mental health workers, public health workers, government officials, recovering addicts, and concerned citizens. *[Article copies available for a fee from The Haworth Document Delivery Service: 1-800-HAWORTH. E-mail address: <docdelivery@haworthpress.com> Website: <http://www. HaworthPress.com> © 2006 by The Haworth Press, Inc. All rights reserved.]*

KEYWORDS. AIDS, barebacking, community action, crystal meth, gay, harm reduction, HIV, HIV prevention, homosexuality, methamphetamine, risk management, risk-taking, safer sex, stigma

Harvey Fierstein: Well, good evening everyone. We are meeting in a different place this time.[1] For any of you that were with us last time, we were at the community center. I thank you all for coming. You are here because you have information we want to hear, and maybe we have a couple of things that you might need to hear. We have a panel of experts, but the real experts are you, because we are asking questions that have not been asked before.

There is a rise in HIV in our community. After 20 some odd years of knowing how to get rid of this disease, we have not managed to so. We need to know why. We need to take care of each other. If we are going to be a community and be responsible as a community, we must be responsible for ourselves and for each other. The government is not looking to take care of us. We need to take care of each other and ourselves. To do that, we need information. To get the information that we all have, we need to share. We are here to all share, learn something, figure out what the right questions are, maybe what some of the answers are. Please, please listen carefully and share what you can. There is a video camera somewhere; when it comes time to share, if you do not want to be taped, simply say, "I don't want to be taped." The camera will be shut off immediately and you have to worry about none of that. Do you all want to make ground rules and then I will introduce everybody? They want to do some "thank you's." Go ahead boys.

Dan Carlson: Thank you Harvey. Good evening. Welcome to the Challenging the Culture of Disease, the Crystal Meth HIV Connection, hosted by Harvey Fierstein. I'm Dan Carlson, and this is Dr. Kellerhouse. We are the organizers of this forum. Let me welcome you here tonight to this second in a series of four forums we are organizing on HIV prevention for gay men in New York City. I would like to also welcome our out-of-town guests from Boston, Washington and Miami and anyone else who has traveled from outside of New York to attend tonight's event. Thank you all for making the trip and being here tonight. Welcome also to our elected officials and representatives of service organizations here in New York City. At the first forum held this past November 16th, more than 300 people turned out to join the public discourse about what is taking place in our community with regard to HIV transmission. Fortunately that dialogue will continue through these forums, due in large part to our sponsors and supporters. I'd like to thank each of them right now.

First a very sincere thank-you and a big dose of gratitude to Harvey Fierstein for supporting our efforts at the last forum and this one. We are very grateful to him for his generosity and time, enthusiasm and spirit. He has played a central role in making these events a success and we thank him so much. He brings a great deal of intelligence, credibility and passion to the discussion. He is not only an activist and an icon, but a leader and a hero. So I want to thank Harvey for being here.

In addition, our sponsors demonstrate, through their support, a deep commitment to HIV prevention and to these events as a powerful, unifying force in which to build community. I would like to thank them now as well. The H. van Ameringen Foundation, Broadway Cares, Equity Fights

AIDS, Callen Lorde Community Health Center, the American Foundation for AIDS Research (AMFAR), and Astor Medical Group. A special thank you to Dr. Kim in Astor Medical Group for gifting us the large posters, which serve as a very nice backdrop for our event tonight.

Many thanks also to our media sponsors, *Gay City News, HX* and *Next,* and some banner space that was offered to us from Gay City News, Gay.com, My Gaydar, Manhunt and Planet Out.

It was clear from the forum held on November 16th that our community yearns for a constructive discussion about rising new HIV infections. In judging by the turnout here tonight, it appears that that hunger is growing and that a dialogue is needed. I think we know in our collective guts that something is wrong. My hope for tonight is that this forum becomes a powerful first step, inspiring change and action. If you are a private citizen and you have come here tonight to express concern, share an experience or offer a solution as it pertains to crystal meth and HIV, then share it. This forum is for you.

This forum is designed for us as private citizens to come together, identify with each other and talk about our experiences with this drug and begin to formulate solutions. Let us use this time to energize each other, and renew our sense of community and support of us taking care of each other better. Complacency from each other in our service organizations can no longer be tolerated when it comes to our health. And now I would like to introduce Dr. Kellerhouse.

Bruce Kellerhouse, PhD: Thank you. When government and non-government agencies, to whom gay men have entrusted their lives, fail to respond effectively to rising rates of HIV infection and crystal meth addiction, they place gay men's lives in jeopardy. When private citizens such as Peter Staley, Dan Carlson and I organize and in some cases pay for HIV prevention efforts (see Appendix Figure 1), something very serious is amiss. We see it around us, in our friends, acquaintance and colleagues. We know that the health and well-being of our community is in jeopardy because we witness it and/or we experience it ourselves and yet we do not talk much about it.

We doubt there are many gay men among us here tonight who have not in some way been affected by crystal meth use in our community. Most of us know someone. Some of us have tried it ourselves or been affected by it in some other way. Yet crystal meth use is one of many shards that form this mosaic that might explain why more men are becoming infected with HIV. Other pieces include the perception that HIV is a manageable disease and that it is no big deal to live with it. Or the widespread use of the

Internet as a private means of finding sex partners and the unexamined practice of bareback sex to avoid plastic sex, either on crystal or off.

In the January issue of *Gay City News*, editor Paul Schindler decried the lack of leadership, among AIDS prevention groups and the gay community, in addressing the alarming news about HIV and crystal meth. This void in leadership poses some important questions. What is the HIV prevention strategy here in New York City for gay men? Where are the public messages that counteract the perception that HIV is now a manageable disease? Where are the public information campaigns that continuously warn us about the dangers of crystal meth use? What are we doing as a community to reinforce behavior that supports staying uninfected? As private citizens, Dan Carlsen and I find the complacency on the part of our leaders troubling and unacceptable. The truth about crystal meth and HIV needs to be told and it is the responsibility of our service organizations to do so. We need their help, and we need their help now.

It is time for us as a community and as individuals to take responsibility for our own health and health of those we love. It is time we change the way we view and create HIV prevention strategies. It is time that we as gay men move from the death-saturated culture of the 1980s, and the disease-saturated culture of the '90s, into a present day culture of wellness, vitality and life. Let us use this time tonight to talk about these difficult and perplexing topics and make substantive change possible. Thank you.

Harvey Fierstein: So here is how we are going to work it. I have a panel here and I am going to introduce each one of them. They are going to make a brief opening statement, after that, we'll have a little bit of a discussion among ourselves. Then we will open up the floor to the room. The only rule is that we do not attack. We are here to build, not attack. So please let us try and remain positive in our attitudes. I am thrilled to introduce this really wonderful panel that the two gentlemen have put together. They have a lot to teach us all.

Peter Staley is up first. He is an AIDS activist since 1987. He is a member of ACT UP and a leader thereof. He was appointed to President Clinton's AIDS task force on drug development. His website, AIDSmeds.com offers comprehensive treatment information for PWA's. He created and financed personally the ad campaign you see there. He is a shining example that we can take power over the world.

Peter Staley: Thank you Harvey. I would like to offer a quick explanation of why I did the ads (see Appendix Figure 2), but before that I would like to thank those publications that have run the ads *for free, including Gay City News, HX, Next, Circuit Noise*, and Boston's *In News Weekly*. I would also like to thank Verizon for its surprising and unsolicited offer to print and place the ads on 20 additional phone booths in Manhattan, starting a few days ago, at their own expense.

Even though I have received most of the credit and blame for the ads, they were co-designed by Vincent Gagliostro, one of ACT UP's greatest political graphic designers. So please give Vincent some credit and blame also. Those six-pack abs aren't his, but they were his idea.

As I mentioned at the last forum with Harvey, I am a recovering crystal meth addict. During my addiction and my continuing struggle to stay clean, I have witnessed a heartbreaking amount of destruction and despair caused by crystal meth. One thing I was not seeing was an outcry about what this drug is doing to our community. The silence was deafening, and not just from our AIDS organizations, but from our city's health department and our gay political leaders as well. The most harmful silence of all was when a few queens dishing the dirt would have a good laugh about somebody being high on "Tina," and nobody else at the table would summon the courage to say, "Are you guys nuts? Haven't you heard what Tina does to people?"

Why can't we all start to speak loudly and consistently about this drug's risks? Why is the gay community uncomfortable about pointing the finger at a party drug that is destroying so many lives? Some have said that demonizing a drug will have no effect on how many people will try the drug. I really wonder if that is true. If you all don't mind, I would like to do a quick poll of the audience. I am going to ask a question that all the democratic presidential candidates have been asked; so if any of you out there are planning to run for president some day, please remember there are cameras in the room. Please raise your hand if you have ever tried marijuana. [raising of many hands, some laughter] That's good. There is a lot of honesty in the room tonight. Now please raise your hand if you have ever tried ecstasy. [raising of many hands] Wow, that's a lot of honesty. That's good. Now please, raise your hand if you have ever tried heroin. [a sprinkling of hands among the audience are raised]

It's a big difference. There must be a reason why we choose some drugs over others. Ask yourself, "Why haven't most of us tried heroin?" It is because we know the risks and we are justifiably scared by those risks. It is not because the government has said, "Just say no!" Nobody is advocating for a wag the finger, "just say no" approach to crystal meth. It is because we have heard about heroin's risks our entire lives in hundreds of ways from friends, family, the mainstream press, movies, TV, documentaries, you name it. If we keep quiet about crystal meth's risks so as not to offend our friends across the table who are having a good laugh about it; or not to offend the sensitivities of some harm reduction advocates; or for fear of handing the Radical Right another club with which to beat us over the head, then countless more gay men will try crystal, thinking it is the new and improved version of ecstasy. Not to mention all the straight men and women who are beginning to party with it as well.

I know we are uncomfortable with having our dirty laundry aired in the mainstream press. Those who hate fags love to brand us as sex-and drug-obsessed, disease-ridden perverts. The issue is perfect ammo for them. So be it. I for one do not fear their hate. We are strong enough as a community to sing about our strengths, of which we have many, while at the same time confronting our demons. Remember when AIDS first hit the mainstream press in the 1980s? It was the perfect ammo for the Radical Right to beat us down. But, instead of cowering in fear, we rose up, we publicly fought back, and every advance the gay rights movement has had since then owes some credit to that moment.

So here we are in 2004, and once again, silence equals death. We need more than a few phone booth ads or a couple of articles in the gay press to fight against the glamorized reputation of a drug that is destroying too many good lives in our community. We need to speak honestly and loudly about the real dangers of crystal meth. We need to provide political cover to our gay leaders and our city health officials who might fear being blamed for stigmatizing gay men if they speak out about this issue. We need their help in this fight. As for tonight, let's try to define the problem, be civil to each other and brainstorm some solutions. Thank you.

Harvey Fierstein: The second panelist is a member of our community who is in recovery. Trevor P. is here tonight to share, briefly, his story with us.

Trevor P.: Thank you, Harvey. Hi, my name is Trevor and I'm 27 years old. A little bit about my upbringing, background, just so you know what one addict looks like. I was raised in New Jersey, in what most would consider a happy childhood: rural, nice parents, horses, cows. I mean drug-free, drink-free all through high school. In fact, I was quite against drugs and alcohol. I went to school to be a public school teacher, went to a public university to be a teacher, and went into a 7-year relationship in college. Once again, mainly drug-free. My only encounter with drugs or alcohol was in college. I tried them, did my thing the first semester or two and put it behind me.

After my 7-year relationship concluded, I had it in mind to live near New York City–because of watching shows like *Queer As Folk.* Or there's this fabulous gay life out there: there's drugs and sex and just about every impulse you can follow. Heck, you know, that's New York I think.

So leaving a 7-year relationship in the suburbs, I moved to Jersey City. That was in February of 2001, I think. I will correct myself if I am wrong. Within 2 months, I had found ecstasy. It just happened upon me and I loved it. I thought, "Okay this is fun. This will teach me something and I will put it behind me when it is done." And about three months later, I had found this drug called crystal. I had heard about it in passing, that people have incredible sex on it. It lasts for hours and hours. I'm like, "Ooh, crystal sounds great." "It sounds interesting." And sure enough, the dealer I was getting ecstasy from happened to sell crystal as well. So at my first encounter with crystal someone, in passing, said, "You know I shouldn't start you on this. It's bad stuff." And I'm like, "I'm a bad boy, you know. I want the candy." That was my warning. My first experience with crystal was July of 2002. It worked for me. The sex was hot and I will say that my first experience using crystal was also my first experience barebacking in a group situation. It was just hot; it was just great. I had barebacked maybe two or three times prior to this, each time sober. But my partner went through a litany of questions that would turn most people off: "Are you negative? Are you this? Are you that? Your favorite color?"

However, my first time on crystal, it just did not matter. It was just hot; all the barebacking fantasies that my generation–somewhat complacent in regards to the AIDS crisis that preceded us–had. I am 27 years old and AIDS has not personally touched me. It has now, but I have not been touched by friends or relatives dying from this disease. So I had in the back of my mind, if it were to happen–not that it would–there are always vitamins you can take. So I kept playing the odds. I would get tested after a crystal binge and going out and playing. I would get tested 6 weeks later and it would come up negative. I would think, "Okay, the odds are going in my favor." And it worked. It was great. I was powerful. I was having fun.

Let's jump ahead from July to November. I was infected–text book infection. I was having unprotected anal sex, and the person came in me, or almost did. Or I think he did. And I said, "What are you doing? Don't do that!" And this was in a sex club where barebacking was the norm. If you asked for condoms, eyebrows were raised. And I had no idea. I just did not understand at the time. I just thought everyone was negative and having a good old time. So this guy finishes and I say, "I'm negative." And he's like, "Well I'm positive." So I get up and I say to him, "No sweat, catcher's call. My fault." I didn't want to make a big deal of it. I said, "Okay, gotta go." In the back of my mind, I'm like, "hmm." Two weeks later, I get a little fever, but it was just a sneeze fever. That was it. In January of 2003, I was diagnosed with HIV. For three months after that, I did not use crystal meth. Getting through medications, getting used to that. I began meds right away. I had trouble. They were not easy to start taking. But once you adjusted, it was fine, I guess.

Within three months I was using again. I thought I would never use, but I used again and the using got more intense. I spent a summer out in Fire Island and had the summer of freedom and love I had always wanted. The crystal usage just kept working and working more and more. And it began taking over. I began to go one night, two nights, three nights. I mean this is a story typical of many, if not most crystal addicts. Eventually it took over my life. I'm thinking of myself, "What kind of son did my mom raise?"

Looking at myself, having HIV, let's skip ahead a year to November of 2003. At this point, my weekends are now 4-5 day weekends. I am bringing drugs to my place of work. I am bringing drugs to a church where I'm a choir director. I had gone there high numerous times. In fact there has been rarely a sober Sunday for a year and a half. One Sunday, I just skipped church and called in sick. I lost a relationship, a boyfriend who just said enough is enough. I decided to celebrate by going out for another four days.

I woke up from all that and realized that something was wrong with me. I did not know the extent of my sickness and what I was battling. I have always considered myself a very self-aware and self-loving person. I do take care of myself quite a bit, and yet I used what I consider one of the most insidious and deceitful and over-glamorized drugs available to gay men. I do not blame crystal meth for my HIV. I am responsible for my disease, and I will tend to myself as an added responsibility for life. It is a complication to my play and my sexual partners. But I hope tonight to add some perspective as to my role when I was playing in the scene and my HIV disclosure to partners. I am in recovery. I have been sober for three weeks and I intend on staying sober for life. I am certainly honored and grateful to be here sharing what I can with you tonight. Thank you.

Harvey Fierstein: Our next guest joins us from across the country. Dr. Steven Tierney is the director of HIV Prevention in San Francisco. He is co-chair of California's HIV Prevention Planning Group. He is a certified addiction specialist and licensed mental health counselor. He is committed to finding solutions that work for real people and getting government to understand what our community needs. Dr. Tierney.

Steven Tierney, EdD: Hi everybody. It is great to see this huge crowd here; it really speaks well of the community. My name is Steven Tierney. I am the director of HIV Prevention for the city and county of San Francisco. I am also a gay man always and an MSM whenever possible. I think that is important. For those of you who do not know that expression,

MSM, that is the way the CDC [Centers for Disease Control] used to classify us when they would study us: *Men Who Have Sex With Men.* In their new evaluation procedures for this year, they have decided to change that to MTM: *male to male sex.*

I came to my work in public health after a long time of community activism and gay and lesbian civil rights work in Massachusetts. There I was head of the state-wide gay and lesbian political organization, back a long time ago when we passed the second in the nation gay and lesbian civil rights bill. So I come to the work in public health not just as a professional in the field of public health, but as a gay man who fought for a long time to open the doors of government so that gay men, lesbians, bisexuals and transgenders could have jobs in government. Because we believed it was important. As taxpayers, we had a right to be heard and to be part of the decision-making process.

So at this point, I think it would be immoral for me or for any of us in public health to turn our well-positioned and well-paid backs on the community and on young people like Trevor who did not have the experience of fighting pre- and post-Stonewall; who did not have the experience of not being able to work in those places; and who did not have the experience, as he mentioned, of watching many around us get sick and die.

Why, I think the question was, aren't public health officials, particularly the gay, lesbian, bisexual and transgender ones, more responsive? I think there are two things going on, neither of which is a good enough excuse. One is that there is still a pink closet in health departments. A couple things happen. One is that you get hired in a health department and there is a certain level to which you can rise as the gay or lesbian point person. If you get tagged as that [a gay person], no matter what your job–even if you are in tuberculosis or restaurant inspection–whenever the community comes, you get trotted out to be the reception for that meeting. While it is all well and good that we have that chance to communicate, it does have an impact on people's careers and on people being taken seriously. So, as Peter mentioned, we need to support those in public health and to remind them that they work in the government, and that they work for us, and that they have a responsibility.

As for the second piece, in San Francisco we got a new ACT UP when the old one expired. The new ACT UP in San Francisco, some of you may know, are people that do not believe that HIV causes AIDS and do not believe that we should do HIV prevention because it puts us in partnership with people who are sex negative and drug negative, et cetera. This group's interactions with folks that worked in the health department were particularly aimed at gay men who worked there and were particularly lively. So the other thing that I think exists in health departments is what we refer to as the "lavender bunker." People have dug in and are trying to stay out of the line of fire of the gay and lesbian newspapers, out of television new shows that call us anti-sex or anti-drug, or that suggest that folks in the health department need to meet with "real gay men" in the community. Which is why in my jobs, both in San Francisco and at the state-wide level in California, I always try to remember, as I said in the introduction, that I am a gay man. I am a gay man who lived through the '70s and '80s. And, like many others, I became an alcoholic and an addict and I have eight years in recovery.

I bring all of that experience to the job and it is the reason that I have a job in San Francisco: as a matter of fact, because of that ability to relate and a personal integrity about relating on a day to day basis as an honest and open gay man in recovery. So I think one of the things that people like me can bring is a real strong message that we need to change the way public health has worked over the last few years. We have had a message that said "AIDS Equals Death." Then, when people stopped listening to that, we rolled out "Hepatitis Is Coming and It Equals Death." And then we rolled out "Syphilis Is Coming and It Equals HIV Which Equals Death." And now we have tried for the last couple years to say, there is this new drug thing and "Drugs Equals Death." Well as the five hundred people in this room right now know, we are not dead. And probably some of us have had sex this weekend and some of use may have done drugs. And if we did not, we know somebody that did and they are not dead. So the message of trying to scare the community into behaving does not work. It has not worked. And, if it ever did, it certainly is no longer appropriate.

We need messages that respond to the realities of our lives. The realities of our lives are that crystal meth is a terrible drug to which people get addicted really quickly. In the course of recovery, which any of you that have had the experience know, there is a relapse factor to crystal meth that has not been properly studied and needs to be. If you know anybody that uses crystal meth as their drug of choice, you know it just kicks your ass. It is a horrible drug for relapse. We do need to talk to young folks and we need to be honest with them. Harm reduction messages are good, but we need to be really, really honest about the potential of this drug to take a really horrible bite out of your life and for the recovery not to be easy at all.

But the fact of the matter is that we try to paint it as just something terrible and horrible. We do not do harm reduction. If funded by the CDC, we are supposed to just say "Don't do drugs. It's a really awful thing and it's terrible for you." Yet young people come to San Francisco for vacation and they get some crystal meth and some Cialis and they have a hard on for 36 hours–which they want. And the first couple of times that happens, it does not seem like such a bad thing in the abstract. We need to give messages that say to people, "You know, that is a temporary high that leads to a permanent long-lasting life of addiction and recovery and is really, really problematic."

So what can government do? There is a problem in government at the federal level, here in New York at the state and city level as well as in California. Our mental health and substance abuse budget in San Francisco is about to be cut by 12-20% and at the state level as well. So the reality is we cannot count on government to respond to this message alone. But as taxpayers, we also cannot let government off the hook. I think government has to be responsible. So in San Francisco, we tried a few things that I would just quickly go through here as possibilities. We used our HIV prevention dollars to fund an outfit called Tweaker.org. If you have not looked there, I suggest that you do. It is a harm reduction website; it gives good information and it encourages people to think about what they are doing and to do it as safely as possible and to get recovery services when they are ready. We have also done needle exchange for a long time in San Francisco by declaring a state of emergency. The Republicans who have run the state over the years do not allow us to do needle exchange unless there is a state of emergency, so every two weeks our board of supervisors declares a state of emergency.

We do most of our work in San Francisco by going out and talking to other members of the community, besides those who work in public health. We have got a new campaign for injection drug users called *Shoot With a Friend,* and it is designed to help people prevent overdose and know what to do about it when it happens. The reason we do these campaigns is because they are needed, and because it says to people in the streets that we have some idea about the real life of people who are using injection drugs. If they can trust us on that, maybe they can trust us when we give them other messages.

We also have funded two organizations in the city, New Leaf Services and Stonewall Project. Because they are substance abuse programs, they should be funded by the substance abuse dollars of CDC in the city. However, they each had a waiting list of 45 days. So again, if any of you have ever done speed or know anybody that did, you can imagine what putting somebody who's actively using speed on a 45 day waiting list, just how useful that might be.

This past year we opened a storefront called Magnet. It is a center for gay men's health and sexuality. It offers in a storefront setting right in the middle of the Castro. It offers HIV and STD counseling and testing and treatment. It offers a variety of other health services, as well as some computer terminals and just a social setting. There is a DJ on Friday nights. It is an opportunity for men to come into a place in the Castro and ask the kind of questions that we ought to be asking. Both Stonewall and New Leaf, the two crystal services that I mentioned, have staff stationed there during all the open hours.

Most importantly, however, what we have done is to have forums just like this one. We have tried on a steady basis to have the subject of crystal meth be in the newspapers, the gay newspapers, on television, the subject of community forums and we have tried to talk to people about what the real issues were. Those of you who have been to San Francisco know that Castro Street is actually pretty small. We have had a large number of young people, ages 18-25 who were homeless and had gotten very much involved with crystal meth. So we decided that it was time to open up a single room occupancy emergency shelter program for them. We pulled together a variety of people from the office of Human Services, from the AIDS office, one of the members of our board of supervisors and a number of community organizations, and we said, "There's a hotel, a single room occupancy hotel that's currently open." We talked to the owner and he said if we were willing to take it immediately, he would be willing to rent out the top floor with 12 rooms for young people on our services. Well I am happy to report, that in 6 weeks, we found 8 young people who the director of human services personally walked through the system to get them made eligible. We got the money together through private and public sources, and this week eight of those young people are now off the street and in emergency housing.

Those of us who are part of the community must demand inside and outside the health department, that there be no more turf wars, no more worrying about where the money comes from, no more worrying about who gets credit for what happened. I think what the community demands, what the community deserves and what this terrible scourge of crystal meth requires of all of us, is to sit down at the tables together or in the auditoriums together. And when we leave the room at the end of the night, have solutions to the problem, not just more discussion; solutions that we insist our public officials deliver within a very reasonable period of time.

When we celebrated Martin Luther King Day recently, I happened to read the letter from the Birmingham jail. If you have not read it in a while, go back and read it. In it, Dr. King very, very powerfully told us that "justice too long delayed is justice denied" and that he was not interested in people telling him to slow down or to be patient. Because if a community that was oppressed waited with patience for the government to respond, it would never happen. So he said there were four things that we must do. One, collect the facts. That is what we are doing here tonight. Two, negotiate with the health departments. They are here tonight and they are listening to you so tell them exactly what you need and what you want. Three, what King calls self-purification, what are we willing to do? Are we willing to do the volunteer work to raise the funds as Peter has done? Are we willing to get out there and do the work? And four, direct action. If the government does not listen, you know where they're at. They work for you. Go and talk to them directly. Thank you.

Harvey Fierstein: The final member of our panel is Steven Lee, MD. Dr. Lee is a psychiatrist in private practice who is on the faculty at Columbia. He has a subspecialty in substance and substance abuse treatment. He is a consultant for Asian & Pacific Islander Coalition on HIV/AIDS (APICHA) and Callen Lorde's–I love this word–psychopharmacological intervention for crystal meth detoxification.

Steven Lee, MD: Thanks. I want to thank everybody for the opportunity to participate in this community forum tonight. It is something that I think is incredibly important, something that I am seeing as an epidemic that's happening here in New York City. For the past 7 years, I have been working closely and doing research with the gay community, in particular with club drugs. I think my most educational experience though has been working off and on with the Callen Lorde Community Health Center since 1999, and seeing what has been happening to our community. It has really been changing since I first started working there.

At first, I would estimate about 10% of the men referred to me for psychiatric evaluation had some kind of issue with crystal. I had to leave for a little while, and by the time I came back in 2002, I would say at least 1 out of every 3 came to me with a crystal problem. And that does not mean that they were coming asking for help with crystal, but that means that they had a crystal problem that significantly affected whatever it was they were coming to see me about, whether it was depression, anxiety, life problems, the crystal itself, hearing voices, paranoia, whatever it might be. And, unfortunately, only a small number of those people had the insight to know that crystal had something to do with the difficulties they were experiencing. But it was quite shocking to see that much of a change between 1999 and 2002.

At the same time at Callen Lorde, we were getting a large number of HIV positive people coming in, through our testing program. Most of these people knew exactly what HIV was, how to prevent it, what they needed to do. Despite all of that, we were still seeing people coming in large numbers and turning positive. The medical director, Dawn Harbatkin, estimates that probably one out of every three people who test positive at Callen Lorde says that they know that crystal meth has something to do with them turning positive. I really see that this as an emergency for our community. So I am very grateful for the opportunity to come and speak with you all about this.

I was asked to come here to talk about the biomedical aspects of crystal, and HIV and how these two things relate to each other. I think it is important to understand the very strong effects that crystal has on the brain in order to really understand why is it so hard to stop using crystal once the addiction has set in. I want to give you a biological framework to develop your opinions, thoughts and ideas about what crystal is doing to our community. The opinions that you voice are going to shape initiatives and policies, and we need to make sure that they are based on factual data and things that we know, not just on passions. I know this discussion is going to be full of a lot of passion today. I am going to keep my discussion as brief as possible and touch on some biomedical aspects. I want to try to reserve as much time as possible for the community discussion, because that is the richest part of what is going to happen tonight.

In addition to the feelings, or the psychological experience that crystal causes, there is a very real biological phenomenon that causes the compulsion to use crystal again and again–even when people have a very strong desire to stop. As you have heard, a lot of people do not want to be stuck on crystal, but for some reason people keep going back to it again and again. In a manner of speaking, the brain becomes biologically hardwired to repeat that behavior. Because this hardwire circuit is part of the same brain circuit that is stimulated in the brain by sexual behavior, we usually see crystal and sex paired together in a very powerful and intimately tangled combination. And here is where the problem with HIV risk comes in. Crystal is different from alcohol and heroin, which may make one a little bit cloudy, a little bit unaware of what's going on, may make one give up the ideas and notions one had about HIV. However, with crystal it is very different. One feels very clear; one's mind is sharp; the person feels great. The drive to do crystal and to have sex is so intense, it gains an overpowering importance. Taking precautions, or even the fear of getting HIV, even though one is aware of its existence, becomes so small, relative to the compelling importance of getting high and having that really, really intense sex.

For people who already have HIV, crystal is still a big problem because it lowers immune function. It increases the ability of HIV to replicate in the body and the brain. It exponentially increases the amount of brain damage that people can get from HIV alone. I think it's extremely important to educate people about crystal meth and HIV. Harm reduction is something that we hear a lot about in working with the gay community around drugs. While harm reduction has some usefulness with many drugs, I do not think it works very well for crystal because it is so addictive.

While harm reduction takes a somewhat removed stance to educate people about how to use crystal as safely as they can, at the same time that counselors are engaging people in this form of treatment, these people are continuing to prime their brains, literally "hardwiring" them. I know I keep saying that word again and again, but that's what they are doing as therapists sit back and take a slow, gentle stance of harm reduction. We say to ourselves, "Okay, I am going to start with a gentle approach, and as this person becomes more and more motivated, at that point, I am going to be a lot more aggressive." The problem is that it may take too long. By the time users actually have some motivation for the therapist to kick in with really aggressive treatment it may be too late. Users may have lost their jobs, their families, their relationships with their friends, or they may have already gotten HIV. So clinicians really have to ask, what is the point at which they want to intervene and be more active?

In addition, the principles of harm reduction rely on rational free will in the users and their ability to weigh risks and benefits. Therapists lay the risks and benefits out for the patients and then pray that eventually the person is going to come up with the right decision; hopefully they are going to come to a rational conclusion, that crystal just is not worth the risk. However, once somebody becomes addicted to something as powerful as crystal, there may really not be much rational thought with which to work. Instead of rational thought, one is confronted with plenty of rationalizations, which is what the hardwired brain uses as excuses to keep repeating compulsive use of crystal. I have seen people become like machines, or like animals that live for the purpose of using crystal or having sex. So what use is a harm reduction protocol when one does not really have much rational material with which to work?

So my message is that education needs to be direct, strong and emphatic; that crystal is dangerous and that the safest way to use crystal is not to use it at all. In my opinion, when someone is already addicted, the best treatment at that point is abstinence. Looking at how this drug works in the brain, I do not think that there is any realistic way for somebody to try to scale it back to moderate, occasional, recreational use. From what I have seen clinically, time and time and time again, is that almost invariably down the road reduced usage accelerates back to a point that it is out of control. So I think the message we give need to be much stronger. This is the message that I hope to pass on to you all today.

Harvey Fierstein: We are going to entertain a couple of questions from the audience shortly. So start thinking about what you want to ask. We have a microphone in each of the aisles. You can line up and start getting ready for that.

I want to ask Dr. Tierney a question. In San Francisco, was there coordination between police, district attorneys and health workers? I mean when dealing with an illegal drug and trying to talk openly about it, you are talking about arrest and all that. It is a very complicated issue. On top of which, we have an election coming up in this country where may be entirely balancing on gay marriages. Is this really the time to tell them [heterosexuals] we got another problem?

Dr. Tierney: In San Francisco, when we put a community forum together, one of the groups of people we wanted to make sure were invited were the folks who run some of our circuit parties and all night rave parties. Several of them came to a meeting. When they left the meeting early, a few of the folks who were dealing with issues in recovery said to us, "You know, it's hard for us to take you seriously as a health department when you're sitting at the table with some of the people who sell the crystal in San Francisco." How seriously can you take [these community forums] if those folks who are selling illegal drug–and everybody knows it– are sitting at the table participating in these conversations like respected members of the community. In point of fact, sad to say, we had not made that connection–that if you throw a party that lasts for three days, it might mean that you know that speed is being sold or has something to do with the profits. So we learned a valuable lesson.

What came out of that was that we held a meeting with the police department and the district attorneys office and invited a whole group of the folks to come back and have a conversation. I don't know about the rest of you who are around my age or older, but we came out of a lived experience where we did not deal with the police or the district attorney unless it was because we had been busted for something. So to sit at the table with them as partners, and to have a discussion was fairly daunting and fairly challenging. However, the reality is that San Francisco is a much smaller geographic community than New York City. Folks there did know who the dealers were, who was selling good stuff and bad stuff, and who was really taking advantage of the young people that were on the streets in the Castro and the south market area. So we had to have a conversation with the police and the district attorney. And they showed up, including the head of the narcotics unit.

We said to them, "Why aren't you doing anything about this? If it was happening on Knob Hill you'd certainly be taking care of it." The response was interesting. What they said was that, because of political pressures in San Francisco, they thought this was a gay community problem–and they did not want to be perceived as antigay by focusing in on the gay community. We said, "Well we think you should do your jobs and prosecute folks who are doing things that are illegal and that are taking advantage of folks in a bad way." They were delighted. They said, "Oh great! So now we can go out and do this and let them know that someone has given us the authority." I had a vision of what the newspaper headline the next day would say in the BAR: "Tierney says Bust the Community."

Clearly, that was not what we wanted; but the experience pointed out to us the real challenge that we have. There are folks who are taking advantage of people with active addiction and other mental illnesses–and there are folks that need to be stopped. But most of us have not had the experience of negotiating and dealing with the police and the district attorney's office in a useful way. So we are trying to pave the way in San Francisco and hopefully you will do that in New York as well, trying to figure out how to form a partnership that's respectful and legal and treats our community to the same rights of protection that every other community has.

Harvey Fierstein: Peter, your ad would say, "I've used crystal and had bareback sex." How closely do you really see those two realities?

Peter Staley: In my personal experience, the "crystal underground," as I called it, is a barebacking community. I encountered very few people who use crystal and condoms. But, that said, I think some have directly criticized the ads for directly tying the two together and saying you can wear a condom when you are on crystal.

There are a lot of other reasons leading to barebacking. All of that is true. In fact, I think we could probably come up with a list of a dozen reasons why there has been a breakdown of the safe sex culture nationally. We need to examine all of them. But, as Dr. Lee pointed out, there is a health difference here. A sober barebacker simply cannot accomplish in a 72-hour period what a meth barebacker can accomplish. The crystal barebacker puts himself and others in far more dangerous situations. To get down and dirty about it, plenty of us have been there: you are just fucked raw by the end of that period. You had that many more partners and you do not sleep. A sober barebacker is going to sleep during that 72-hour period. From a health standpoint, just the quantity and the type of sex one is having is far, far riskier. So it is a factor in HIV transmission.

Harvey Fierstein: I've got 30 questions to ask these gentlemen. But it is time to open it up to the audience, so maybe I'll get some of the answers.

Audience Member 1: I'm a psychiatrist working at a hospital-based HIV Clinic. In the last 2 1/2 years in my practice, we have seen an explosion of crystal meth use and it is pretty frightening. As Peter Staley said, there are probably a dozen reasons why there has been a breakdown in terms of barebacking which I also think also has to do with crystal. In terms of the patients I see, there are a whole host of reasons why people are using. In addition to, as Dr. Lee said regarding the psychological addiction, what I found is that many people use crystal with sex as a way of escaping; a way of not feeling; a way of taking oneself out of oneself.

Some of the issues that we [as a community] need to address are issues around mental health, whether it be depression, anxiety; or one that people do not seem to be talking about: homophobia. I still have a lot of guys coming to me from ages 20-50 who use drugs as a way of feeling good about who they are, of feeling okay about being a sexual being. People mention what is happening in terms of marriage. It is great that we are able to talk about gay marriage in the press, but the message given to gay people from those opposed–that their relationships are not valid–is pretty shitty. So I think a lot of these things do contribute to the crystal addiction.

Audience Member 2: I work for the New York City Department of Health and Mental Hygiene. I am also an openly gay man who's HIV+ and a member of our community extremely concerned about the impact of crystal meth use on the gay male community. Two years ago, I resided in West Hollywood. On Friday and Saturday nights, late into the night, you could hear the sirens of emergency vehicles as they rushed to the homes of many gay men who had overdosed on crystal meth. This is an extremely serious danger to our community. On behalf of Dr. Thomas Frieden, Commissioner of the New York City Department of Health and Mental Hygiene, I'd like to share the following comments with you:

> The Department of Health and Mental Hygiene commends you on your efforts to bring greater attention to the issue of crystal meth, particularly as it relates to the increased risk of HIV transmission. The department recognizes that crystal meth use is a growing and serious problem in the gay male community and that it is directly related to increased risky sexual behavior and transmission of HIV and other sexually transmitted diseases. We know that crystal meth use among gay men in New York is growing and that it is correlated to higher rates of HIV and syphilis. Clearly there is a need for increased surveillance, increased education, increased prevention and treatment services. We need to de-glamorize the drug and stress the health implications in terms of increased risk of HIV transmission as well as other negative health impacts, such as

increased blood pressure, accelerated heart rates, anxiety, paranoia and sometimes psychosis. We should advise people that when the drugs effects wear off, users can become depressed, even suicidal. The Department of Health and Mental Hygiene will develop health education materials on crystal meth to be distributed to gay establishments and community-based organizations within the gay community. We currently have an initiative called, Healthy Man's Night Out, which brings health services, immunization, HIV testing, referrals to gay men in gay bars and clubs and gay male venues. In this initiative, we provide education, and make referrals to meth treatment. In addition we will explore ways of expanding this very successful program to emphasize the dangers of crystal meth use and abuse.

Lastly, the New York City Commission on AIDS, a commission established by Mayor Bloomberg, has identified the increased use of crystal meth among gay men as a major risk factor contributing to HIV infection. The HIV Prevention Planning Group will provide a forum on crystal meth as an emerging issue. The DOHMH Office of Gay and Lesbian Health will assume the lead for coordinating an ongoing response to this issue within the department. We will also meet with the San Francisco Department of Health and discuss their initiative. We very much support your responsiveness to this public health issue and we will work with all of you to prevent crystal meth from endangering and destroying the much-valued lives of gay men in New York City. We want you to know we are your partners in this fight.

Audience Member 3: I am a nurse-clinician with a NYC Hospital's HIV satellite clinic. I am also a recovering crystal meth addict myself. I have 7 1/2 months of recovery time. I mentioned both of those facts just to let you know that I have some personal as well as professional experience with this entire problem. I am happy that somebody from the city is actually here and read a statement, but I would chasten him against actually using adjectives like successful programs in advance of the program succeeding. I really appreciate this forum, and everybody's remarks. I think that even if crystal meth were not a major vector for transmission of HIV, crystal meth is an enormous problem in the gay community that in and of itself needs to be solved. If everybody uses condoms and does not pass on crystal meth, we have still got a fucking big problem if everybody is a fucking crystal meth addict. There is no such thing as harm reduction with crystal meth. I appreciate that it has been said, but I am going to reiterate it: there is no such thing as harm reduction with crystal meth. It is impossible, and the damage that it does to our lives and to our community makes that really clear every day.

A speaker before me mentioned homophobia and internalized homophobia. I think they play a big part in this. I also think the pornography industry plays a role in the glamorization of the self-image of what it means to be a gay man. Where does that self-image come from and what are we compensating for when we try to live up to that image? I also think that the damage and loss that we've experienced over the last 20 years as a community, because of the AIDS crisis and this gaping spiritual wound that we suffer, is an enormous factor in everything that we are experiencing here as a community. I believe that as we go forward and try to formulate some methodology to solve our problem, that we need to take into consideration these factors.

Peter Staley: I just want to put my two cents in about this argument about approach to treatment, abstinence versus harm reduction. For those of you in the audience who do not know what harm reduction means–or abstinence, for that matter–the good news is that there are a lot of treatment options for people who are suffering from this drug. There are lots of abstinence-based programs like Crystal Meth Anonymous. There are a lot of meetings every week. There are counseling programs that head more toward the harm reduction approach at GMHC and at the Center, etc. So just reach out and try something. But abstinence based programs basically say the goal has to be to be to stop the drug forever, stop drug use and all drug use forever. Harm reduction is a catch-all for all the other programs that do not have that as a set requirement, but try to just reduce the harm that is occurring from current drug use.

I personally am not anti-harm reduction. I think it can be a very useful bridge for the meth addict. When I first realized that I had a problem, I was still very much in love with the drug. So I sought out a shrink. I asked around for a shrink who was an expert in addictions with gay men and I went into his office and I said, "I've got a problem. I'm doing this a lot more than I want to do it." Then I told him, "The goal I want in working with you is to figure out how to do this less. I want to do it once every three months, and I want you to help me to figure out how to do that." And of course, it turned out to be a crazy idea. But if he were an abstinence-only fanatic, he would have thrown me out of the office and I would have had no help. Instead he said, "Alright, I actually have never heard of anybody being able to control this, but I will work with you on this." And for 9 months, we basically tried harm reduction. And harm was reduced during those 9 months. I did use less, and eventually I came to realize though that the only way I was going to save myself was to abstain. So for a period of the work, it was a great bridge. One thing I can say about harm reduction is that these approaches meet people where they are at the moment. Instead of just saying, "Come back to us only when you're ready mentally to say, 'I'll never use again.'" So I wish the two communities could support each other and work together and not fight against each other, because we need all the help we can get.

Dr. Steven Lee: I just wanted to add to what Peter was saying, which is that I agree that there is too much tension between two really polarized groups, and that both models really do have their merit. Probably the greatest merit of harm reduction is that it maintains the patient alliance or the alliance with the person who is trying to stay in recovery. People who are too far on the side of the abstinence-based model do tend to alienate users and throw them into a place where they do feel isolated and by themselves. People may find themselves faced with an abstinence-based system that judges them, criticizes them, and commands them to do something. I think there needs to be a middle ground where one meets the person where they are.

Audience Member 4: I have worked in harm reduction for the last 12 years, and I am really glad to hear what people are saying. There has always been a middle ground. Harm reduction and abstinence area not incompatible. They are different parts of the same thing, which is to stay working with people. That is what concerns me, Peter, when you talk about demonization and stigmatization, which I think are almost inevitable. They come with the cultural package. However, what I see is that during the bulk of the AIDS epidemic, stigmatization of heroin use, which you said kept people in this room from using, also guaranteed that the half of the infections in New York City–which occurred among heroin users– basically did not matter to most people. The prevention programs were not important to most people. To this day, the funding for those programs has been flat since 1994. During the time [Mayor Rudolph] Giuliani was in office, there was no support coming from the city. Now that there is a little bit of support coming from the city, we actually see that there is a rivalry between the city and state and that they do not talk to each other. Literally, the people working in harm reduction at the state and the people working in harm reduction at the city will not talk to each other. But that is not even about harm reduction, that is about the rivalry between the city and state over who is going to be in control of AIDS funding.

These are the kinds of things we as a community are going to have to address. However, I think it is important to consider, when you talk about stigmatization and demonization, that essentially what you are saying is, that a group of people out there, the ones who will continue to use crystal, the ones who will actually be at risk are the ones who will not matter. Whereas the ones who do matter are the ones who are not demonized, who are not stigmatized because they are not using. I've been working for 12 years with people who are getting locked up and people who are homeless. Harm reduction is not telling them, "Look, your drug use has made you homeless, your drug use has caused you to be locked up." They are coming to me and saying, "My drug use has made me homeless; my drug use has caused me to be locked up." And they are still using. So let's be real about the role that stigma and demonization play. I do not think there is anything wrong with your poster. Frankly, I think it is kind of funny and it is kind of true. But do we want the same things to happen to people who use crystal as use heroin? Do you want them to get locked up? It is kind of racist, to say that, frankly. Anyway, so that's the deal.

Audience Member 5: I am a program director for a needle exchange program. Somebody touched on the idea that there is a harm reduction camp and an abstinence camp. We are all part of the same camp. Harm reduction can include abstinence, and for some people that is the goal. So I want to make sure that is one of those myths that is erased. Harm reduction is also a gateway for many people to go into treatment. One of the differences between harm reduction and a lot of other program services is that it's non-judgmental. It does not stigmatize the user. It stigmatizes the drug, but not the user, and that is a very important point in terms of reaching people.

Our harm reduction center provides mental health counseling, stress management services, case management and a lot of other services that people do not think about when they think needle exchange program. That is another myth, that we only do needle exchange. It is a comprehensive program and it is very important to do it that way. The other thing that we have to also consider is that hepatitis and other blood-borne diseases and sexually transmitted diseases are also on the rise. We only talk about HIV, but we have to also take into account these other diseases.

Finally, our harm reduction center has been trying for the last year to expand our services to reach other parts of the city. There have been some problems along the way which have to do with getting community support for us to do that. As many of you know, the history of needle exchange in New York City has been one where many community members do not want us in their back yard. So that is one area where we could use support. The other is funding so we could hire more staff in order to develop services that extend into other areas, specifically around the meth epidemic. So I am putting it out there for anyone who has any ideas, anyone who wants to work with us, anyone who has any contacts in the Community Board in particular, to help us open those doors so we can reach out. Thank you.

Harvey: Thank you very much. We really do need to keep the comments short because a lot of people want to share. I know there are important organizations here as well, but we cannot turn this meeting into advertisements for organizations. Once again, this is not an attack, but it is a public forum. Please.

Audience Member 6: Someone I love very much right now is in a huge fight with crystal. Many other people I know are. This particular person, we do not know if he will win. But we know that I cannot help him and that hurts both of us. It is a terrible drug. And HIV is a terrible illness. But, in his fight, one thing that he has kept is the sanctity of protected sex. I think that is the issue that is the crux of all of what we are looking at here.

Audience Member 7: I am with a group that does harm reduction for non-injecting drug users, and because of some friends of mine who have had this problem, I have been very concerned about it. I knew about it in San Francisco, before it got here. It seems to me we always knew this about this, though. In the 60s, we came up with something, the "speed kills" campaign. Maybe we just have to put graffiti on the walls again to say speed kills, because this is not just a gay problem. This is the hugest drug problem in rural America. Dr. Lee, what psychopharmacologic treatments do you have for crystal?

Steven Lee, MD: This is a very new field. Unfortunately, there has not been a lot of research done in that area. I'm actually working with Callen Lorde in developing a detoxification protocol that will help people with the very painful process of stopping when they are in a crystal cycle. That is one of the things that sets people up so that they use it repetitively, sometimes on a daily basis for months, because they are terrified of crashing when they stop. We have developed a detox protocol that helps to ease the pain of actually stopping, because some of these people are very highly motivated to quit. So that is one of the things that we do, and it is based on a protocol that has nothing to do with crystal or other stimulants, but it helps them to get off.

In addition, there are some other medications that theoretically can help to decrease some cravings. For some people, those medications help, by boosting the dopamine that crystal methamphetamine depletes in the brain. In addition to that, as has been mentioned by a number of people today, sometimes crystal use can be actually treating something else; so finding out what that something else is going to be crucial in helping that person. Whether it is depression, anxiety, or core issues about self-esteem–some of those are therapy issues some of them are medication issues. But those are also crucial to treat to make sure that somebody does not relapse.

Audience Member 8: I really struggle with these forums in the sense that I think so many incredibly intelligent and passionate people come and leave bereft of next steps. I have dedicated a lot of my professional life to an organization and to HIV prevention. With this kind of gathering of folks who have so much to offer to their communities, I would hate for people to leave not thinking about what they individually can do. So I would like to hear from the panel about that. I would like to offer that there are many spaces we can fill, that crystal is filling in our lives, that we are not filling with alternatives and with conversation. My hypothesis is that crystal fills a need to connect between each other, men and men connecting to each other. Crystal is helping men do that in a very negative and disastrous way. Until we start to talk to each other in the social networks in which we move and in the places that we go, like Allegria next week or the Black Party in March, as volunteer teams or as individuals on our collectives in our own social networks, we need to have these conversations. And I'm very curious to hear from the panelists, what can we do?

Harvey Fierstein: I don't think that anybody who gets into one of these conversations leaves bereft of ideas. I know that in theaters all over New York, minds were changed, discussions were had, and behaviors were changed. So even on the simplest front–where I am working on an ad campaign right now, Peter went ahead with his ad campaign–I really think that airing these sort of things and getting our minds working and empowering our community is what is important here. The organizations that are now in place and have been in place for 20 some odd years have not ended this crisis. Obviously we need more answers and we need more things to be done. I'm thrilled that you are in the community and that you're working towards AIDS reduction but honey, it ain't working! So we need to keep throwing out more ideas. I'm thrilled that Mathilde Krim is sitting here. I'm thrilled that the head of Broadway Cares is sitting here. But the strongest thing we can do is open our minds and share with each other all the ideas, and nobody will leave this room the same way they came in, unless they close their hearts that way. But I'd like to have other people answer that question.

Steven Tierney, EdD: I challenge everybody here, when you go to for your next cup of coffee and you see somebody sitting by himself, talk to him. It is that simple to start it. Find out if he is connected, especially if he is a younger person in our community. Find out if he has just moved here, if he is connected to social services at the [LGBT Community] Center. That might sound a little too simple but it is really not. We know that the most effective thing in fighting adolescent addiction is to be connected to somebody. So we do not have to join organizations and pay dues, although that is a great thing. We can start very personally, where you go for coffee or where you go for lunch, talk to somebody who is sitting by himself or herself and make sure that they are connected somehow to social services and health care in New York.

Dan Carlson: You touched on the exact purpose of this event. You know, there is a lot of silence out there. A lot of people are not talking about this. We organized this forum so we can come together, share our experiences and then, hopefully, people will take this conversation, what they hear here, what they learn here, and go back and talk to other people. A lot of people came up to me after the first forum and said we were just talking about that in our office or amongst our friends. That is exactly what this is about, as Harvey said, empowering people to go out and talk to people in their social networks about this. Then hopefully that will translate into conversations with their partners.

Audience Member 9: I am a social worker in private practice, largely with gay men. I see a fair number of people with crystal use seroconversion, and it seems to me it is linked with the idea of connection. It is a human thing, not a gay thing, to feel seen, to feel desired, to feel very close to somebody. Sex is that kind of relationship. You know where you are just pressing flesh and you are just right next to somebody and there is this intense bond. I guess I see it. I come from a mental health point of view and I think if we question what people are really getting with these relationships, that might be a good place to start. Because I think there is a lot of approval around sex. And sex is great. But if you're going there and your need is to feel really connected with somebody, to feel intimate, and you're getting a 30 second ass-fucking or something out of a line of 50 people, that is not really what the fantasy is.

Harvey Fierstein: I think it sounds hot. I'm sorry, when I hear a straight line I have to do the joke.

Audience Member 9: I'm not straight.

Harvey Fierstein: The joke was, maybe not for you.

Audience Member 9: Anyway, I guess an examination of these things would be useful, and more conversation in the community. I think therapy is a good way to figure out what the real emotional needs are behind a lot of the crystal, the sex, the sexual compulsion, and a lot of seroconversion.

Trevor P.: I would like to add that when I was first infected, I took a three-month hiatus from using, just from the shock. My first time going back to using, I went to the same sex club where I was infected. It was really emotionally bewildering as I am walking up the steps and going through the whole thing. I am there talking and in a conversation with one of the regulars. I say, "I'm positive now." And he says, "Welcome to the club." And I just realized, my eyes opened up, that was what it was about. This particular venue was catcher's call; there's no lifeguard on duty. Everyone watches out for themselves and sometimes people do not.

Sometimes people are too uncomfortable to talk about their positivity and will just fuck you unprotected and come in you. And then you ask them if they are clean and they will say, "Oh yeah, yeah, yeah, yeah." But they are not. In terms of the belonging, I just wanted to connect with that. That it is very much like an exclusive club. In a way that is what helped my usage increase. Now I'm positive, well this is the one thing I can do now. I have my passport to decadence. I don't have to worry about it anymore. So you know what? I am just going to use and use and it just does not matter. It is a very unhealthy "belonging-ness" that the culture is stuck in. I was very much a part of it. I had my member's card. It is cut up now, but I was there.

Stephen Lee, MD: You are asking some very important questions about what is going on even before someone gets to the crystal. The crystal is treating something lying underneath. What you say is true, that a lot of people would probably benefit from therapy. Unfortunately the majority of the kids, the young people that are out there are not going to be able to get to therapy. The community has to ask itself, what are we going to do to address these core issues of low self-esteem, of poor self-acceptance, of difficulty exploring sexuality? All of the things that get instantly cured with crystal. "I feel great about myself. I am wonderful. I can have sex like I always wanted to, and I don't have to be afraid of it anymore." What can we do as a community for these young people that can actually help them? I put that out there without any answers for you, but it is a really important question.

Audience Member 10: I do holistic health and life coaching with mostly gay men, many of whom are in recovery. We have touched on connection, self-esteem and working with people and understanding how to get to harm reduction or abstinence. But also wondering where things begin. I think that we have a responsibility as a community, club promoters, whomever. When kids come to New York City they are drawn to the allure of the sex and the fun. You open the *HX* magazine and you see the beautiful bodies, and you see Roxie. Well, why doesn't Roxie have a night talking about crystal and its dangers? Come out and dance and learn about the dangers of unprotected sex. Here's the danger with crystal. Why don't we have those kind of evenings, instead of "here's the new CD and here's the great new dance re-mix"? Here's a night about crystal, and here's how it's going to destroy your life.

We all have a responsibility, I think. Whether it's HX magazine or the ads promoting the beautiful bodies, it is about learning to love yourself. Not nurture your ego, but nurture yourself from the inside. I think the kids who come to New York have been very depressed in their small towns. I was born elsewhere, and I was not really accepted when I was there. I came to New York to like go, go, go and sex was fun. But I learned that you really have to love yourself. I do not think that a lot of young people have that knowledge. In addition to just reducing the harm, how can we have kids come together in a community forum? Here is how you can love yourself more; here's a dance; here's something else we can do.

Audience Member 11: I'm with Soulforce New York, but I am mostly here as a concerned community member. I've lived in New York for 20 years and this forum has really shown me how factionalized the community has become. When I first got to New York, there were community meetings that we had at the firehouse in Soho. We met and there were lesbians, black people, everybody. It was really a community-based group and we were all together because we were different. We were happy we were different. Now it has just become so factionalized it seems to me that we are really not talking to each other. People are so alienated, and we have to speak out.

I think, there was this prohibition against telling someone who was positive that it was not acceptable to give it to somebody else, to have unsafe sex with somebody else, because the big AIDS organizations thought that would stigmatize people who were positive. But when I hear friends of mine who do that, I just say it is not really acceptable if you know you are positive and you are doing that. I think we need to start having consciousness-raising groups. We do need to start speaking to each other again about our different experiences. What it is to be a lesbian, what it is to be a black gay man, what it is to be a white gay man, and to really talk about those things. Because this is really not magic, it's just what is happening. It is really an epidemic.

The last thing I want to say is I really hope we have learned from the AIDS epidemic not to build more alienating community-based organizations that are mostly worried about funding. So I really hope that we do not go to the police and that we really do start to talk to each other.

Audience Member 12: I work for the harm reduction coalition. This forum is great. I do not think those posters or this forum are going to change anyone or stop anyone from using crystal tonight or any other time. But what it is doing right now is making us all talk about drugs. Drugs and alcohol have affected the lesbian and gay community more adversely than the straight community for years and we have never talked about it. It has never been addressed. Now we have a crystal epidemic. This is the opportunity. If we do not take it, we are blowing it.

As someone mentioned, drugs go in cycles. This is not the first cycle of speed. It is also not the only cycle that is going on in this country right now. The changing community norms come from drug users. Drug users do it themselves, that is why the "speed kills" campaign of the 60s actually slowed down the use of speed amongst people in the 60s and 70s. That is the way it is going to happen here. People do not wake up in the morning and say, "I'm going to go out and find a social service agency to go and visit today." They wake up with a hangover; they wake up depressed. The conversations have to happen out there. It has got to be in the coffee shops. The message has got to be on the sides of buses. It has to be the community talking about it.

Audience Member 13: Hi, I am from Miami. Right now, crystal meth is just touching South Beach. So you are our models of how we are going to attack it once it comes to South Beach. It is in South Beach, but not as bad as in New York. It is not in the clubs, it is in private parties. It is in our bathhouses. It's also on the Internet. We have a cyber outreach program and it is actually working. Right now we are trying to get an evaluation piece; we are trying to get more funding for cyber outreach. I love Peter Staley's ad because it speaks the truth. Dr. Tierney, I came up with [the slogan] *Meth Equals Death* because there's one thing nobody's talking about and that is how many domestic violence issues have come up because of methamphetamine use. See the movie *Tweaked* and you will see how many children, how many spouses, and how many significant others have been affected by this drug.

Audience Member 14: I am a writer and I've done a hell of a lot of crystal since the year 2000. I went to a support group because I wanted to be off the roller coaster, and the lady asked me, "How long you been clean?" It reminded me of growing up gay down south when I was 15 and I told everybody I was gay and they said things like I was dirty. So my point is, we have to move beyond the question of "How long have you been clean?" "Since I took a shower this morning," was my response.

Whenever you ask how long someone has been clean, it implies that drug use makes them dirty. Being gay made me dirty, or being HIV positive made me dirty. Being clean is not a scientific, clinical diagnosis. So I went right back to crystal after that support group.

Audience Member 15: The way I have really been affected by crystal is I had to live with a girl who was a crystal addict who had an abortion on my toilet. She does not live with me anymore and she is still using. I do not know where she is. I wish her well.

I work in a gay bar in Chelsea. I've worked there for 6 years. I am from the South as well where there were not that many things for gay people to do. I have worked in a gay bar to support my artistic career. For 6 years, I have worked in a bar serving men who are trying to connect and who only connect under the effect of a substance, be it alcohol or be it crystal or be it cocaine or anything else. And I am saying I love Peter Staley's ad as well, and I find it very interesting. It has affected so many people, whereas when Sound Factory runs an ad on the back page of *Next* called Sound Factor Raw, for men who love men, at $60 a pop, not one eyebrow is raised.

I would just like to say that you need to raise yourself up and preach by example. Even a simple thing like a yoga class has to be nude for some gay men to take it in Chelsea. I would just like to say there's more to life than sex. There is more to life than sitting at your fucking computer and trying to hook up. My only plea here tonight is for business owners, people who are wealthy, people who have a business, people who own a restaurant, a nightclub, open your doors to people to come in free of charge and connect.

Audience Member 16: I am a psychopharmacologist and also a psychiatrist. I would like to echo everyone who pointed out that there are important issues of self-esteem and what it means to grow up in this society with a queer identity, and the impact it has on all sorts of challenges we face. But I do not think that we are going to engender an evolution of society here in this room. Secondary to the institutional developments in the wake of HIV in the 80s, there was an evolution in our community, but that was secondary. That was not planned. We cannot sit around and wait to engender self-esteem in all those who are lacking it in order to stem the tide of this. I think we have to go directly to the guts of the issue.

Not all, but much of the discussion tonight has been about treatment opportunities for people who are already having problems with crystal. Of course it is important that we focus on that. However, similar to the early days of HIV, we also have a massive opportunity here to try to stem the tide of those who have not yet been exposed. And as always, Peter goes straight to the point immediately when he compared the circumstance to how other people feel about different other drugs. Heroin is essentially demonized in our culture, at least in certain strata of our culture, and that is why so many of us have never gone near it even though we have gone near other drugs. We have to do the same thing with crystal. I think that is where the largest bang for the buck is, to do something to demonize crystal at the level that stops entry into the problem.

Audience Member 17: I am an actor and not involved in any organization. I love these ads. This the first time I've seen ads of this type in New York City, really linking crystal and HIV together. I want to compare them to the ads and the giant media campaign I remember as a high school senior in rural New England, where they reached me on how to stay HIV negative. In the late 80s and early 90s, they worked all of those ad campaigns from many different media angles, like Madonna on MTV. Everyone came together with the same message, different strategies on it and different routes to it, but how to stay negative, how to protect yourself. Those ads worked.

I know that we in New York enjoy a special position. We create the media, that is true. I think that if everyone here recognizes this as a legitimate and serious problem, we can prevent other young men from coming from elsewhere into New York, and then becoming infected because they simply did not know the danger. I know that Trevor P. mentioned that his dealer said it was bad, but perhaps it was only his dealer that said it was bad. If that is the only one voice you hear saying it is bad and every other voice in the media you hear says "This is great, this is wonderful," you discount that one, because we all synthesize all the media that we receive. Because it was the fact that I was bombarded as a teenager, I knew how to keep myself negative during the early and mid-90s. I think that's where we need to go with this. Thank you.

Harvey Fierstein: I think there is an interesting thing coming up out of our comments. Do we demonize crystal meth or do we demonize HIV? Which are we more frightened of and what is the connection?

Audience Member 18: My experience with crystal meth was with my best friend whose ashes I just had to throw into the Hudson River last week. We used to party with crystal together. I basically tried it because he introduced me to it. I was curious, but because I did not like the burning sensation in my nose, I stopped doing it. It was that simple. But I would hang out with him and we would go to parties together.

But with this tragedy that just hit me, I felt like I was thrown back 20 years ago. The thing I have to say is that I think the reason why I am standing here today is because I have been able to find a way to fill a spiritual void in my life. I am a Buddhist and I think that that is something that really helps to keep me here today. I open my home every month once a month to invite friends and fellow gay Buddhists to have a dialogue creating a sense of self-worth or just encouraging each other to really realize that we all are very special. No matter who we are or what background we come from, or what we do in our spare time, we are all special individuals. And that has grown now into a bigger forum. We did one at the [LGBT] Community Center recently that was very successful. But I just wanted to say that I think that it is important for us to try to find a way to have a strong sense of self, self-worth, self-esteem. Whether it is Buddhism or whatever spiritual journey you have to take, find some way to realize the value of your life. Then we will not have to deal with these terrible destructive issues in our community.

Audience Member 19: I want to thank you all for having this forum. I think the ad is really great. I think it makes a very clear point. I think another common link people have been touching on in different ways is sex addiction, which is also really, really rampant in the gay community. I think that that is something that we really cannot talk about. I think people are used to talking about being addicted to a drug, and it is almost kind of trendy to be addicted to a drug. But people are still very uncomfortable talking about sex addiction. I think our gay culture glorifies sex to an absurd degree. But I think that may be a subject for another forum.

Audience Member 20: I am one of the young folks that you are referring to and I thank you for extending the invitation to come up and talk. The connection thing is really a key; it has been touched on a lot. I had a really great experience growing up gay. I am from Long Island. I was passing through all the really excellent resources that they had for gay youth there. That has been wonderful. But everywhere I go, the young men I try to connect with, it is difficult. I think you may not remember how difficult it is. One solution is to volunteer. Any agency that works with gay folks would love to have you. Think of all the connections that you can make, and you will love it.

Harvey Fierstein: Remember, we also have a Community Center. If you want to start a group to introduce people, we've got everybody there like Sage [Senior Action in a Gay Environment]. We've got everybody, so our Community Center is a great place to connect.

Audience Member 21: I am in the early stages of recovery from a crystal meth addiction. I wanted to speak because I wanted to put a minority face on this discussion. I feel that one of the reasons why many hands were not raised when the audience was asked about the use of heroin is because the room was not filled with the people that often come under the stereotype of being a heroin user. Crystal meth has a different race association and if you were in some of my recovery meetings, if that racial group was there, many more hands would be raised. I think that is something that you might want to acknowledge. My suggestion is that the strength that I am gaining from my recovery is definitely due to analyzing why I was sad before I started using. It is definitely what I have to return to in moments of temptation, to remind myself. My suggestion would be to analyze and demystify the body type that is actually in the ad's photo. I think what would create the inclusion is to analyze why butch, white and muscular has become the ideal of what is desired in our community. I have personally suffered serious bouts of low self-esteem because I am black, thin and femme. So I have felt I have felt very far from that.

Audience Member 22: I am an addict. And when I came into recovery, they told me that I needed to stay away from people, places and things. What that meant was that I had to leave the gay community, which was a very sad day for me. I couldn't have that, so I moved to New York City and I found a lot of sober, safe places. The Center was probably the safest place when I was trying to get sober and clean from drugs. I believe that what keeps people away from drugs is some facility, some, some connectedness 24 hours a day. Most treatment facilities, unless you are an inpatient, are not 24 hours a day. I needed to talk to people 24 hours a day because I wanted to use 24 hours a day. I used 24 hours a day, and I have not used now in 22 years.

Audience Member 23: I also remember dancing at the firehouse. I think a lot of important issues have been brought up. One thing that I think we learned the hard way from HIV prevention is you cannot have one size fits all. I think there are motivations for using crystal that are different for men who are seropositive and men who are seronegative. In trying not to drive a wedge in our community between those who are positive and those who are negative, we fail to be able to deliver messages and services and support that are tailored to the different needs of those people.

What we do know about, what little behavioral research has been done, we know that men who are positive are using crystal to have sex, men who are negative are using crystal to connect. That does not mean that there are not some correlations there, but unless you address those things on their own terms, I do not think you're helping anyone.

Harvey Fierstein: I just want to thank you all for your candid comments, for coming, for caring, for being part of our community, and please, please, stay in touch with each other and us. Thank you.

NOTE

1. An earlier, standing room only public forum on barebacking was held on November 16, 2003 at the GLBT Community Center in New York City.

APPENDIX

FIGURE 1

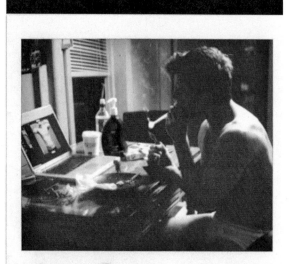

FIGURE 2

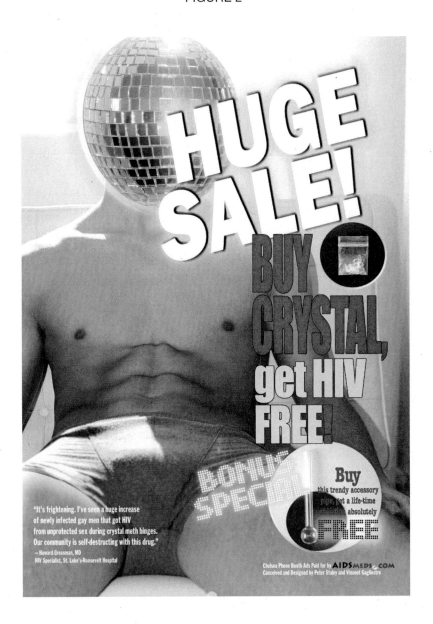

Crystal Meth Testimony

Peter Staley

SUMMARY. The author provides a personal account of crystal meth-amphetamine addiction. He describes the difficulties and treatment experienced by someone who is gay and an AIDS community activist. The author describes his first encounter with crystal meth, the consequences of using it, treatment strategies he found helpful, and, from the patient's perspective, what clinicians can do to prevent and treat crystal use. *[Article copies available for a fee from The Haworth Document Delivery Service: 1-800-HAWORTH. E-mail address: <docdelivery@haworthpress.com> Website: <http://www.HaworthPress.com> © 2006 by The Haworth Press, Inc. All rights reserved.]*

KEYWORDS. Abstinence, addiction, AIDS, anal intercourse, club drugs, cocaine, crystal meth, harm reduction, gay men, HIV, homosexuality, men having sex with men (MSM), sexual risk taking, treatment, unsafe sex

Thank you for this opportunity to speak about this relatively new healthcare crisis among gay men in New York City. I have spent most of my adult life fighting AIDS, including some very empowering, wonder-

Peter Staley is the Founder of AIDSmeds.com; *editors@aidsmeds.com.*

Address correspondence to: Peter Staley, 135 Eastern Parkway, #13G, Brooklyn, NY 11238.

[Haworth co-indexing entry note]: "Crystal Meth Testimony." Staley, Peter. Co-published simultaneously in *Journal of Gay & Lesbian Psychotherapy* (The Haworth Medical Press, an imprint of The Haworth Press, Inc.) Vol. 10, No. 3/4, 2006, pp. 45-47; and: *Crystal Meth and Men Who Have Sex with Men: What Mental Health Care Professionals Need to Know* (ed: Milton L. Wainberg, Andrew J. Kolodny, and Jack Drescher) The Haworth Medical Press, an imprint of The Haworth Press, Inc., 2006, pp. 45-47. Single or multiple copies of this article are available for a fee from The Haworth Document Delivery Service [1-800-HAWORTH, 9:00 a.m. - 5:00 p.m. (EST). E-mail address: docdelivery@haworthpress.com].

Available online at http://jglp.haworthpress.com
© 2006 by The Haworth Press, Inc. All rights reserved.
doi:10.1300/J236v10n03_03

ful, yet tragic years being one of the leaders in ACT UP (AIDS Coalition to Unleash Power) then TAG, the Treatment Action Group.

I have also fought for gay rights, including our sexual liberties. And I have enjoyed those liberties, and delighted in our community's ability to enjoy a good party.

But now, sadly, some gay men have taken things too far. We are partying ourselves to death and despair. We have chosen some poison to party with, called crystal meth, and it is systematically destroying the lives of thousands of gay men. It is directly killing a few. It's helping many others become HIV positive, and it is making thousands of us addicted for life, with all the wreckage addictions can cause.

I should know. In New York, crystal meth started becoming the gay community's party-drug *du jour* in the year 2000, and that is when I gave it a try. The drug's reputation was, until recently, simple–try it, and you will have the best sex of your life. For many gay men, this reputation is irresistible.

The first time I tried crystal meth, I snorted one bump, less than $5 of the drug, which kept me high for a 12 hour sexual marathon. The second time I tried it, I smoked it. I needed twice as much to stay high during the first 12 hours, and I kept partying for 48 hours, with no food, multiple sex partners, no condoms, no discussion of HIV status, no worries, just sex. I lost 10 pounds, mostly from dehydration, by the time I was finished.

This is the typical crystal meth sex binge, although they can frequently last for three, four, or even five days. I became addicted to the drug almost immediately, and it took me over two years of recovery programs, with frequent relapses, before finally getting clean. I am happy to report that I have been sober for over 18 months.

I would like to discuss quickly what helped me to get sober. After the first couple of binges, I was completely in love with crystal meth. I bragged to a good friend about my sexual exploits on the drug. He was a fellow AIDS activist, and he had actually heard about how risky crystal meth was, and how it destroyed lives. He told me this bluntly. I was furious at him for raining on my parade, but he planted a seed of doubt in my head.

I think this allowed me to recognize my addiction earlier than I would have otherwise. Most guys have a prolonged period of denial about what crystal is doing to their lives. In fact, they think it's the only good thing in their lives.

In my case, being told bluntly, early on, that meth was a highly addictive substance helped shorten my period of denial.

The first thing I did was seek out a good shrink with a reputation for helping gay men with addictions. However, I was still madly in love with the drug, so I told my new shrink that what I needed was help in controlling my use of the drug. In other words, at this point, I was only ready to hear a harm reduction message.

He, like my friend, was also blunt. He told me that he worked with lots of guys who have a problem with meth, and he had never met a person who learned to control their crystal meth use. He then went on to say that maybe I would be the first, and he was willing to help me. In other words, he told me the truth about meth up front, but did not kick me out the door when I wasn't buying it initially. He planted more seeds.

Eventually, after 9 months of trying harm reduction methods, I came to realize that my friend and my shrink were right–that I could not control this drug–that I had to stop for good. I started an abstinence-based program, relapsed many more times, and eventually entered an out-patient program–the Realization Center on Union Square.

After thousands of dollars of group and individual therapy, thankfully partially paid for by my insurance plan, I am finally sober, and I've got a great life again.

If I can give only one word of advice to those of you who are the front line defense against the crystal meth epidemic, to those of you who are healthcare workers that might hear the early confessions, or notice the early signs of addiction, it would be this: be honest with us about the risks of crystal meth, even if we are not ready or willing to hear it. You will plant a warning seed that will help us get past the denial a little quicker. There are ways to be honest about meth without lecturing and alienating your patients. I know it is hard, but remaining silent because you are uncomfortable with the subject, or worried about offending your patient, should not be an option. We need your honest diagnosis of what this drug might do to us.

All of us–healthcare workers, friends, AIDS organizations, gay organizations, gay leaders, politicians, the city's department of health, and the press–must speak loudly and bluntly about the risks of crystal meth. As we used to say in ACT UP, silence equals death. I, for one, will no longer remain silent about the destruction this drug is causing. I hope you will join me.

Thank you.

Medical Complications
of Crystal Methamphetamine

Antonio Urbina, MD

SUMMARY. This article reviews available literature on the medical morbidities associated with methamphetamine abuse in HIV-infected patients. Medical complications include hypertension, hyperthermia, rhabdomyolysis, and stroke. One fatal case of ingestion of methamphetamine with HIV medication has been documented. Two fatal cases of ingestion of HIV medication with the amphetamine analogue n-methyl-3,4 methylenedioxymethamphetamine (MDMA, or "ecstasy") have also been reported. Some molecular researchers suggest that dopaminergic systems are vulnerable to the combined neurotoxicity of HIV infection and methamphetamine. Methamphetamine is a new challenge related to treatment and prevention of HIV infection. *[Article copies available for a fee from The Haworth Document Delivery Service: 1-800-HAWORTH. E-mail address: <docdelivery@haworthpress.com> Website: <http://www.HaworthPress.com> © 2006 by The Haworth Press, Inc. All rights reserved.]*

KEYWORDS. AIDS, cardiovascular, drug interactions, HIV, HIV dementia, medical complications, methamphetamine, neurotoxicity, neurotransmitter toxicity, side effects, substance abuse

Antonio Urbina is Medical Director, HIV/AIDS Education and Training, Saint Vincent's Hospital HIV Center, 170 West 12th Street, NR 1413, New York, NY 10011.

[Haworth co-indexing entry note]: "Medical Complications of Crystal Methamphetamine." Urbina, Antonio. Co-published simultaneously in *Journal of Gay & Lesbian Psychotherapy* (The Haworth Medical Press, an imprint of The Haworth Press, Inc.) Vol. 10, No. 3/4, 2006, pp. 49-55; and: *Crystal Meth and Men Who Have Sex with Men: What Mental Health Care Professionals Need to Know* (ed: Milton L. Wainberg, Andrew J. Kolodny, and Jack Drescher) The Haworth Medical Press, an imprint of The Haworth Press, Inc., 2006, pp. 49-55. Single or multiple copies of this article are available for a fee from The Haworth Document Delivery Service [1-800-HAWORTH, 9:00 a.m. - 5:00 p.m. (EST). E-mail address: docdelivery@ haworthpress.com].

Available online at http://jglp.haworthpress.com
© 2006 by The Haworth Press, Inc. All rights reserved.
doi:10.1300/J236v10n03_04

MEDICAL COMPLICATIONS

The short term effects of methamphetamine (MA) are protean and are mediated primarily through the release of large amounts of dopamine (DA) and smaller amounts of norepinephrine (NE). This can lead to tachycardia, hypertension, tachypnea, hyperthermia and central nervous system excitation effects similar to those induced by acute cocaine ingestion (Lynch and House, 1992). MA toxicity can also lead to rhabdomyolysis and cardiovascular events (Albertson, Derlet and Van Hoozen, 1999). One 5-year retrospective review of California emergency department admissions with a final diagnosis of rhabdomyolysis reported that 43% had detectable urine levels of MA (Richards et al., 1999). Cardiovascular responses elicited by binge administration of MA include vasoconstriction, vasculitis and focal myocyte necrosis (Varner et al., 2002).

Cardiopulmonary events from chronic MA use are well documented and include myocardial infarction and stroke. These potentially devastating events usually occur in relatively young patients. Four cases of stroke associated with MA use in patients ranging in age from 29-45 years have been documented (Perez, Arsura and Strategos, 1999). Smoking of MA has been associated with acute pulmonary hypertension and dilated cardiomyopathy (Hong, Matsuyama and Nur, 1991).

MA may also have immunomodulatory activity, particularly by impairing CD8-mediated cytotoxic T-lymphocyte function (House, Thomas and Bhargava, 1994). This may be of clinical importance in primary HIV infection as CD8 activity is responsible for early suppression of lentiviral replication and viral set point (Bagasra and Pomerantz, 1993).

Long term MA abuse also results in bruxism and periodontal disease (Venker, 1999; Richards and Brofeldt, 2000) increasing dental costs in one prison study by 200 percent (Weland, 2002). Illicit MA may also be contaminated with multiple harmful byproducts. Acute lead poisoning has been reported and presents with anemia, encephalopathy, myalgias and hepatitis (Buchanan and Brown, 1988).

METABOLISM

MA and related compounds, including dextroamphetamine and n-methyl-3,4 methylenedioxymethamphetamine (MDMA or "ecstasy") are metabolized by the CYP2D6 isoform of the cytochrome P450 enzyme system. The genetic polymorphism associated with the P450 system results in significant individual differences in responses to these compounds (Ramamoorthy, Tyndale and Sellers, 2001). For instance, 3-10% of the Caucasian population is deficient in CYP2D6 and may be at increased risk for MA toxicity (Brosen and Gram, 1989)

DRUG INTERACTIONS BETWEEN MA AND ANTIRETROVIRALS

Fatal interactions between amphetamine analogs and protease inhibitors (PI) used to treat HIV infection have been recently reported. Protease inhibitors are metabolized primarily by the CYP3A4 isoform and also inhibit, and in some cases induce this enzyme in varying degrees. The PI ritonavir can also affect three other P450 enzymes including CYP2D6. As ritonavir has greater affinity for this enzyme than either MA or its analogs, concomitant administration may result in 3-to 10-fold increases in either MA or MDMA levels (Pritzker et al., 2002). Delavirdine is partially metabolized by CYP2D6 and may have similar pharmacokinetic interactions with amphetamines.

A case report from Australia documents an HIV infected patient on a combination of stavudine, saquinavir and ritonavir who died after injecting MA. Toxicology reports showed MA levels of 0.5 mg/l, consistent with MA overdose (Hales, Roth and Smith, 2000). Two case reports document fatalities following ingestion of ritonavir containing regimens and MDMA (Henry and Hill, 1998; Baker and Bowers, 1997).

NEUROTOXICITY

MA's neurotoxic effects are the most devastating and potentially permanent medical sequelae of its chronic abuse. Studies in rats indicate that MA accumulates in the brain, with a brain to plasma ratio of 10 to 1 (Melega et al., 1995). This, coupled with the long plasma half-life of approximately 12 hours, probably accounts for the majority of central nervous system toxicity.

NEUROTRANSMITTER TOXICITY

MA causes neurodegeneration in the dopaminergic and the serotonergic nerve terminals in animals (Woolverton et al., 1989). Human studies provide evidence that MA use leads to a reduction of dopamine transporter (DAT) levels, which are a marker of dopamine cell terminals. One study of 15 HIV-negative MA abusers studied with positron emission tomography (PET) scans found significant DAT reductions. Subjects had used MA for up to 11 years, and were abstinent for at least 2 weeks before the PET scans. This was associated with neuropsychiatric testing evidence of impaired motor function and impaired verbal learning. DAT levels fell within the range seen in low-severity Parkinson's disease in three of the subjects. Although impaired on tests of both gross and fine motor speed, extrapyramidal symptoms were not seen. Investigators hypothesized that this was due to the relative youth of the subjects, whose mean age was 32 (Volkow et al., 2001b). It is not known whether these DAT reductions reflect irreversible DA terminal damage or neuroadaptive changes that may recover with protracted abstinence. Another study of five former MA users showed that although DAT levels recovered significantly with abstinence of 12-17 months, neuropsychological function did not. Neither the gross nor fine motor speed tests improved significantly, nor was there improvement on the Rey auditory verbal learning test (in which subject has to learn and recall lists of unrelated words) (Volkow et al., 2001a).

SYNERGY BETWEEN MA AND HIV

The clinical features of HIV dementia are those of a subcortical type, including: psychomotor slowing, apathy and memory deficits. In advanced HIV dementia, symptoms such as bradykinesia, altered posture, gait, and incontinence can occur (Berger and Arendt, 2000).

The etiology of HIV dementia is poorly understood, but it is a metabolic encephalopathy that involves both brain cell loss and neuronal dysfunction. Supporting neuronal cells (such as microglial cells, macrophages, and astrocytes) induce damage by secreting inflammatory substances that damage or kill brain cells. Neurons themselves are not infected with HIV (Nath, 2002; Minagar et al., 2002).

Experimental evidence suggests the HIV-1 viral proteins gp 120 and Tat are toxic to DA neurons (Nath et al., 2000a; Nath et al., 2000b). There is overlap in that both MA and HIV target DA neurons. HIV affects the DA neurons in subcortical structures, particularly the basal ganglia (Lopez et al., 1999). MA targets DA in many regions of the brain, including the orbitofrontal cortex (thought to be implicated in impulsive behavior) as well as the dorsolateral prefrontal cortices and the amygdala

(Sekine et al., 2003). Some researchers have proposed that the underlying mechanisms for the neurotoxicity of combined HIV infection and use of MA, suggest that dopaminergic systems are most vulnerable to such combined neurotoxicity (Nath et al., 2002; Nath et al., 2001; Grant et al., 1999).

Researchers found that exposing feline astrocytes infected with feline immunodeficiency virus (FIV) to MA increased FIV's ability to replicate and mutate by 15-fold (Gavrilin, Mathes and Podell, 2002). These findings imply that MA use in patients with HIV could increase the prevalence of HIV brain disease (HIV Associated Dementia, Minor Cognitive Motor Disorder) in patients not on ARV's. This awaits verification in human studies.

CONCLUDING REMARKS

MA has serious acute cardiovascular effects that may interact with HIV medications to cause increased toxicity or death. Neurological complications resulting from dopamine depletion can result in irreversible neuropsychiatric symptoms, including memory loss, and may be synergistic with HIV-related dementia symptoms. Psychiatric morbidity in MA abusers with HIV infection includes acute psychotic reactions and long-term depression. MA abuse represents a new medical challenge in HIV treatment.

REFERENCES

Albertson, T.E., Derlet, R.W. & Van Hoozen, B.E. (1999), Methamphetamine and the expanding complications of amphetamines. *Western J. Medicine*, 170:214-219.
Bagasra, O. & Pomerantz, R.J. (1993), Human immunodeficiency virus type 1 provirus is demonstrated in peripheral blood monocytes in vivo: A study utilizing an in situ polymerase chain reaction. *AIDS Rev Hum Retroviruses*, 9:69-76.
Baker, R. & Bowers, M. (1997), Ritonavir and Ecstasy. *BETA*, Mar:5.
Berger, J.R. & Arendt, G. (2000), HIV dementia: The role of the basal ganglia and dopaminergic systems. *J Psychopharmacology*, 14(3):214-221.
Brosen, K. & Gram, L.F. (1989), Clinical significance of the sparteine/debrisoquine oxidation polymorphism. *European J. Clinical Pharmacology*, 36:537-547.
Buchanan, J.F. & Brown, C.R. (1988), "Designer Drugs": A problem in clinical toxicology. *Medical Toxicology & Adverse Drug Experience*, 3:1.
Gavrilin, M.A., Mathes, L.E. & Podell, M. (2002), Methampehtamine enhances cell-associated feline immunodeficiency virus replication in astrocytes. *J. Neurovirology*, 8:240-249.

Grant, I., Heaton, R.K., Dawson, L.K. & Marcotte, T.D. (1999), Abuse of methamphetamine and cocaine may enhance HIV associated neurotoxicity. *Archives Clinical Neuropsychology*, 14(1):130.

Hales, G., Roth, N. & Smith, D. (2000), Possible fatal interaction between protease inhibitors and methamphetamine. *Antiviral Therapy*, 5:19.

Henry, J.A. & Hill, I.R. (1998), Fatal interaction between ritonavir and MDMA. *Lancet*, 352:1751-1752.

Hong, R., Matsuyama, E. & Nur, K. (1991), Cardiomyopathy associated with the smoking of crystal methamphetamine. *JAMA*, 265:1152-1154.

House, R.V., Thomas, P.T. & Bhargava, H.N. (1994), Comparison of immune functional parameters following in vitro exposure to natural and synthetic amphetamines. *Immunopharmacology & Immunotoxicolology*, 16:1-21.

Lopez, O.L., Smith, G., Meltzer, C.C. & Becker, J.T. (1999), Dopamine systems in human immunodeficiency virus-associated dementia. *Neuropsychiatry, Neuropsychology & Behavioral Neurology*, 12(3):184-192.

Lynch, J. & House, M.A. (1992), Cardiovascular effects of methamphetamine. *J. Cardiovascular Nursing*, 6:12-18.

Melega, W.P., Williams, A.E., Schmitz, D.A., DiStefano, E.W. & Cho, A.K. (1995), Pharmacokinetic and pharmacodynamic analysis of the actions of D-amphetamine and D-methamphetamine on the dopamine terminal. *J. Pharmacology & Experimental Therapeutics*, 274:90-96.

Minagar, A., Shapshak, P., Fujimura, R., Ownby, R., Heyes, M. & Eisdorfer, C. (2002), The role of macrophage/microglia and astrocytes in the pathogenesis of three neurologic disorders: HIV-associated dementia, Alzheimer disease, and multiple sclerosis. *J Neurological Sciences*, 202(1-2):13-23.

Nath, A. (2002), Human immunodeficiency virus (HIV) proteins in neuropathogenesis of HIV dementia. *J. Infectious Diseases*, 186(Suppl 2):S193-198.

Nath, A., Anderson, C., Jones, M., Maragos, W., Booze, R., Mactutus, C., Bell, J., Hauser, K.F. & Mattson, M. (2000a), Neurotoxicity and dysfunction of dopaminergic systems associated with AIDS dementia. *J. Psychopharmacology*, 14(3): 222-227.

Nath, A., Haughey, N.J., Jones, M., Anderson, C., Bell, J.E. & Geiger, J.D. (2000b), Synergistic neurotoxicity by human immunodeficiency virus proteins Tat and gp120: Protection by memantine. *Annals Neurology*, 47:186-194.

Nath, A., Hauser, K.F., Wojna, V., Booze, R.M., Maragos, W., Prendergast, M., Cass, W. & Turchan, J.T. (2002), Molecular basis for interactions of HIV and drugs of abuse. *J. Acquired Immune Deficiency Syndromes*, 31(Suppl 2):S62-69.

Nath, A., Maragos, W.F., Avison, M.J., Schmitt, F.A. & Berger, J.R. (2001), Acceleration of HIV dementia with methamphetamine and cocaine. *J Neurovirology*, 7(1): 66-71.

Perez, J.A., Jr., Arsura, E.L. & Strategos, S. (1999), Methamphetamine-related stroke: Four cases. *J. Emergency Medicine*, 17:469-471.

Pritzker, D., Kanungo, A., Kilicarslan, T., Tyndale, R.F. & Sellers, E.M. (2002), Designer drugs that are potent inhibitors of CYP2D6. *J. Clinical Psychopharmacology*, 22:330-332.

Ramamoorthy, Y., Tyndale, R.F. & Sellers, E.M., (2001), Cytochrome P450 2D6.1 and cytochrome P450 2D6.10 differ in catalytic activity for multiple substrates. *Pharmacogenetics*, 11:477-487.

Richards, J.R. & Brofeldt, B.T. (2000), Patterns of tooth wear associated with methamphetamine use. *J. Periodontology*, 71:1371-1374.

Richards, J.R., Johnson, E.B., Stark, R.W. & Derlet, R.W. (1999), Methamphetamine abuse and rhabdomyolysis in the ED: A 5-year study. *American J. Emergency Medicine*, 17:681-685.

Sekine, Y., Minabe, Y., Ouchi, Y., Takei, N., Iyo, M., Nakamura, K., Suzuki, K., Tsukada, H., Okada, H., Yoshikawa, E., Futatsubashi, M. & Mori, N. (2003), Association of dopamine transporter loss in the orbitofrontal and dorsolateral prefrontal cortices with methamphetamine-related psychiatric symptoms. *American J. Psychiatry*, 160(9):1699-1701.

Varner, K.J., Ogden, B.A., Delcarpio, J. & Meleg-Smith, S. (2002), Cardiovascular responses elicited by the "binge" administration of methamphetamine. *J. Pharmacology & Experimetnal Therapeutics*, 301:152-159.

Venker, D. (1999), Crystal methamphetamine and the dental patient. *Iowa Dental J.*, 85:34.

Volkow, N.D., Chang, L., Wang, G.J., Fowler, J.S., Franceschi, D., Sedler, M., Gatley, S.J., Miller, E., Hitzemann, R., Ding, Y.S. & Logan, J. (2001a), Loss of dopamine transporters in methamphetamine abusers recovers with protracted abstinence. *J. Neurosciences*, 21:9414-9418.

Volkow, N.D., Chang, L., Wang, G.J., Fowler, J.S., Leonido-Yee, M., Franchesi, D., Sedler, M.J., Gatley, S.J., Hitzemann, R., Ding, Y.S., Logan, J., Wong, C. & Miller, E.N. (2001b), Association of dopamine transporter reduction with psychomotor impairment in methamphetamine abusers. *American J. Psychiatry*, 158(3): 377-382.

Weland, M. (2002), Crook's bad teeth costing taxpayers. *Kootenai County News*, Jan 20.

Woolverton, W.L., Ricaurte, G.A., Forno, L.S. & Seiden, L.S. (1989), Long-term effects of chronic methamphetamine administration in rhesus monkeys. *Brain Research*, 486:73-78.

Methamphetamine Emergencies

Paul L. DeSandre, DO

SUMMARY. The alarming rise in emergency department visits related to crystal methamphetamine use is cause for concern for any clinician caring for patients who may use the drug. According to the most recent Drug Abuse Warning Network (DAWN) report, the problem is escalating in New York City in particular. The toxic effects of the drug can be dangerous and even fatal. Early recognition and basic interventions can be life sustaining, so it is important for clinicians to understand the range of toxicity and basic management strategies.

There are a number of case reports showing that nearly all organs of the body are affected by crystal methamphetamine use, but certain patterns are clear. Patients may present to emergency departments dangerously psychotic, having seizures, strokes, or heart attacks. Also, patients may be in respiratory distress from asthma-like bronchospasm or may develop kidney failure from the toxic effects of muscle hyperactivity. The disinhibition and impulsivity associated with the frequent combination of methamphetamine and sildenafil (Viagra) puts the individual at serious risk for many sexually transmitted infections, including HIV,

Paul L. DeSandre is the Associate Residency Director of Emergency Medicine at Beth Israel Medical Center, New York, NY; Assistant Professor of Emergency Medicine at the Albert Einstein College of Medicine, Bronx, NY; and Chair of the New York Gay and Lesbian Physicians.

Address correspondence to: Paul L. DeSandre, DO, Associate Residency Director, Department of Emergency Medicine, Beth Israel Medical Center, First Avenue @ 16th Street, New York, NY 10003 (E-mail: pdesandr@bethisraelny.org).

[Haworth co-indexing entry note]: "Methamphetamine Emergencies." DeSandre, Paul L. Co-published simultaneously in *Journal of Gay & Lesbian Psychotherapy* (The Haworth Medical Press, an imprint of The Haworth Press, Inc.) Vol. 10, No. 3/4, 2006, pp. 57-65; and: *Crystal Meth and Men Who Have Sex with Men: What Mental Health Care Professionals Need to Know* (ed: Milton L. Wainberg, Andrew J. Kolodny, and Jack Drescher) The Haworth Medical Press, an imprint of The Haworth Press, Inc., 2006, pp. 57-65. Single or multiple copies of this article are available for a fee from The Haworth Document Delivery Service [1-800-HAWORTH, 9:00 a.m. - 5:00 p.m. (EST). E-mail address: docdelivery@haworthpress.com].

Available online at http://jglp.haworthpress.com
doi:10.1300/J236v10n03_05

syphilis, and antibiotic resistant staphylococcal skin infections. In addition, if a patient is having cardiac chest pain and does not reveal that they are using Viagra, standard emergency care is dangerous. Protease inhibitors, taken by a large number of patients with HIV, may cause a fatal reaction with methamphetamine even after a single dose. Finally, patients requiring emergency care are often in crisis and may be more receptive to intervention. When the decision is made to discharge the patient from the emergency department, a "brief intervention" strategy is effective at establishing that a problem exists, preventing future risk, and beginning recovery. *[Article copies available for a fee from The Haworth Document Delivery Service: 1-800-HAWORTH. E-mail address: <docdelivery@ haworthpress.com> Website: <http://www.HaworthPress.com> © 2006 by The Haworth Press, Inc. All rights reserved.]*

KEYWORDS. Brief intervention, cardiovascular, emergency department, HIV/AIDS, methamphetamine, psychosis, protease inhibitors, pulmonary, sexually transmitted infections (STIs), sildenafil

Crystal meth (methamphetamine) use in New York City is on the rise. In addition to the devastating manifestations of addiction, methamphetamine can cause acute and sometimes fatal medical problems. Methamphetamine may affect nearly all organs in the body; most importantly the brain (psychosis, seizures, and stroke), the heart (acute coronary syndrome or heart attack), the kidney (kidney failure), and lung (bronchospasm or respiratory failure). Some gay men have unique risks with the recent popularity of combining crystal meth with sildenafil (Viagra). The combination increases the likelihood of unsafe sex with multiple partners, leading to an unusual prevalence of sexually transmitted infections (STIs), including HIV, in patients who would otherwise not likely expose themselves to that risk. Also, the combination of crystal meth and Viagra may create a potential danger in treatment for the patient in the emergency department (ED) if the medical staff is unaware of what the patient has taken. Furthermore, protease inhibitor drugs, a common prescription for patients living with HIV, carry a potentially fatal risk when combined with methamphetamine. Clinicians should recognize when emergency care is needed and understand the medical risks of using crystal meth. It is also important to utilize the emergency situation to effect change. Intervention and referral can be more effective in crisis situations and provide a unique opportunity to begin the recovery process.

WHO ENDS UP IN THE EMERGENCY DEPARTMENT?

The Drug Abuse Warning Network (DAWN) Report of July 2004 noted a 54% increase in methamphetamine related emergency department (ED) use from 1995-2002. In New York City, the increase was 82%. Over 60% of emergency department visits also involved other drugs, the most common being marijuana, alcohol, and cocaine. The likelihood of under reporting and incomplete recognition makes this trend particularly disturbing.

Nationally, the DAWN Report describes the majority of methamphetamine patients coming to the ED as white (65%), male (58%), and ages 18-34 (>50%) (DAWN Report, 2004). One study looked at 461 patients over 6 months presenting to their ED with confirmed methamphetamine use. The patients tended to be Caucasian males, arrived via emergency medical services, more likely to have sustained trauma, and were more likely to be admitted to the hospital (Richards, Bretz et al., 1999).

PSYCHOSIS AND ACUTE RENAL FAILURE

Both the addictive "rush" and the many medical problems associated with it are due to methamphetamine causing a prolonged excess of stimulatory (sympathetic) neurotransmitters, primarily dopamine and norepinephrine. This may result in a variety of neurological effects ranging from agitation to frank psychosis. The muscle hyperactivity normally associated with methamphetamine use can escalate into an agitated or psychotic state. This probably accounts for the majority of cases who require emergency care (Derlet et al., 1989; Richards, Johnson et al., 1999). The heavy release of myoglobin from the muscle tissue during such severe hyperactivity is known as rhabdomyolysis. Myoglobin is toxic to the kidneys in high concentration with prolonged exposure. This is one of the most important concerns in methamphetamine toxicity because renal failure can be prevented with appropriate and timely treatment, including sedation and fluid hydration (Richards, Derlet and Duncan, 1998; Henry, 2001).

HEART ATTACK, STROKE, LUNG, AND LIVER

Heart attack and stroke are the most likely causes of sudden death after using methamphetamine (Kalant and Kalant, 1975). Methamphetamine increases heart rate and blood pressure sometimes to dangerous levels. It may cause heart attack or stroke in a patient otherwise not at risk. The irritability to heart and brain tissue can cause fatal rhythm disturbances or intractable seizures, respectively (Varner et al., 2002). Sudden surges in blood pressure may cause direct mechanical injury to blood vessels causing rupture and bleeding (hemorrhage). In the brain, this can result in a devastating hemorrhagic stroke (Mohlesi and Corbridge, 2003).

Methamphetamine use is also known to cause inflammation in blood vessels (Rumbaugh et al., 1971; 1976). This inflammatory response encourages clot formation, leading to inadequate blood flow (ischemia) and possibly tissue death (infarction). This may manifest in the heart as acute coronary syndrome (including heart attack), and in the brain as stroke. Accordingly, one emergency department study found an unusual prevalence of acute coronary syndrome in young patients without cardiac risks, presenting with chest pain after methamphetamine use (Turnipseed et al., 2003). There are also a number of case reports of stroke in young patients using methamphetamine (Rothrock, Rubenstein and Lyden, 1988; Perez, Arsura and Strategos, 1999).

Similar vascular damage may explain other organ involvement such as lung and liver (Jones and Simpson, 1999; Kamijo et al., 2002). Also, crystal methamphetamine is commonly smoked, exacerbating both acute and chronic lung injury and may induce acute bronchospasm (Wolff and O'Donnell, 2004).

Sedation is the primary treatment for the cardiac and neurologic concerns, as with agitation and psychosis. The chemical effects of the sedating medications help decrease heart rate, blood pressure, and seizure activity. One very important difference is that ß-blockers, such as metoprolol, are often used to control heart rate in patients with cardiac chest pain. With methamphetamine and related drugs, ß-blockers have a paradoxical effect on blood pressure and may dangerously exacerbate high blood pressure (Albertson et al., 2001). Other medications, such as phentolamine (an α-blocker), are a safer choice in this setting. In addition, use of sildenafil (Viagra) is a contraindication to the standard treatment of nitroglycerin in patients with cardiac chest pain (Cheitlin et al., 1999). It is important for emergency personnel to be informed of all drugs that a patient has taken to assure proper care.

SEXUALLY TRANSMITTED INFECTIONS

The neurostimulatory effects of methamphetamine induce a sense of power and disinhibition, which in combination with sildenafil (Viagra) may manifest in unprotected sexual activity with multiple partners during a binge period. Patients may present afterward with sexually transmitted infections (STIs), including syphilis, HIV, and antibiotic resistant staphylococcal skin infections (Centers for Disease Control, 2000; James, 2003; Urbina and Jones, 2004). As with any unknown possible exposure to sexually transmitted diseases, patients should be offered Post Exposure Prophylaxis (PEP) for HIV, gonorrhea, chlamydia, and hepatitis B immunoglobulin. Also, patients should be tested for syphilis and Hepatitis B and C, and appropriate follow up should be arranged. Finally, patients should be offered HIV testing and appropriate counseling (Moran, 2000).

PROTEASE INHIBITORS

Protease inhibitors are particularly dangerous in combination with methamphetamine. Both methamphetamine and protease inhibitors are metabolized by a shared enzyme. Protease inhibitors have a much greater affinity for the enzyme than methamphetamine and its analogues. This slows the methamphetamine metabolism up to ten times. The physiologic effects then become extreme, such as uncontrolled blood pressure, extreme temperature elevation, or seizures, and can be fatal with even a single dose of crystal meth (Hales, Roth and Smith, 2000; Harrington et al., 1999).

SAFE DISPOSITION AND BRIEF INTERVENTION

A patient presenting in serious mental or physical condition will likely require hospitalization. For those being discharged from the emergency department, clinicians may often fail to consider the circumstances that caused the individual to require emergency care in the first place. At the time of discharge from the ED, having experienced a medical crisis, the patient is unusually receptive to addressing a drug or alcohol problem. The requirement of emergency care as the result of recreational drug use is often enough to convince a patient of a problem, whether or not the patient acknowledges an addiction. This is an important opportunity for the clinician that should not be missed. One very simple and effective approach for the emergency care provider is the "Brief Intervention." Most of the literature supporting brief interventions in the emergency department is related to alcohol use, but many addictions have common principles guiding intervention and recovery (D'Onofrio and Degutis, 2002). This approach encourages an empathetic yet unequivocal communication with the patient confronting the drug or alcohol problem, and the circumstances that lead to their needing emergency care.

One method to help the clinician remember the brief intervention strategy is the mnemonic, E-D-D-I-R-E-C-T (Empathy-Directness-Data-Identify willingness to change-Recommend action/advice-Elicit response-Clarify/confirm action-Telephone referral) (National Institute on Alcohol Abuse and Alcoholism, 1995). It begins with communicating concern for the patient's well being. Then the patient is provided evidence of a problem as observed by the clinician. If the patient is ready to accept help, they are offered a recommendation for action right away. If the patient accepts, then the details are reiterated and information is immediately provided. If the patient already has a therapist, the patient should be encouraged to contact the therapist, even from the ED, to discuss what happened to them. If the patient does not have a therapist, they should be referred to one as soon as possible. Whenever possible, the follow-up arrangements should be made before the patient leaves the ED. There are several good referral options in New York City and elsewhere, many accessed through the internet, for recovery from crystal methamphetamine addiction (see Referral Resources in Appendix). There are also opportunities to participate in research protocols geared toward facilitating recovery. In considering physician referral for general medical care, the clinician should consider addiction specialists and physicians sensitive to sexual and gender orientation.

CONCLUSION

In our efforts to provide optimal care for those affected by crystal methamphetamine, we should consider whatever opportunities we are given to minimize injury and create possibilities for safe recovery. We know the situation is escalating, so clinicians must be vigilant in encouraging early entry into healthcare.

Recognizing a possible methamphetamine emergency can minimize injury by engaging prompt and safe intervention. The approach in the emergency department may be as simple as fluids and sedation, but some medications could be dangerous to the patient if emergency healthcare providers are unaware that the patient is using methamphetamines or other drugs. It is therefore critical to encourage honesty about any drug or prescription use for anyone requiring emergency care. Also, patients living with HIV must be made aware of the lethal danger of using crystal meth while taking protease inhibitors. Finally, there is a serious risk of engaging in unsafe sex associated with crystal meth use. It is therefore important to assure that both clinicians and meth users are aware of this risk and the time-sensitive opportunity for Post Exposure Prophylaxis (PEP).

The majority of patients presenting to emergency departments are discharged to their familiar environment. Many of those who come to the emergency department as a result of crystal meth use will also likely be discharged. With these patients, it is particularly important to focus on the moment prior to discharge. A few minutes of clear communication with a definitive plan can have a profound effect.

REFERENCES

Albertson, T.E., Dawson, A., de Latorre, F., Hoffman, R.S., Hollander, J.E., Jaeger, A, Kerns, W.R. 2nd, Martin, T.G. & Ross M.P. (2001), TOX-ACLS:Toxicologic-oriented advanced cardiac life support. *Annals Emergency Medicine*, 34(4 suppl): S78-90.

Centers for Disease Control and Prevention (2000), Outbreak of syphilis among men who have sex with men–Southern California. *Morbidity & Mortality Weekly Report*, 50(7):117-20.

Cheitlin, M.D., Hutter, A.M. Jr., Brindis, R.G., Ganz, P., Kaul, S., Russell, R.O. Jr. & Zusman, R.M. (1999), Use of sildenafil (Viagra) in patient with cardiovascular disease. *Circulation*, 99:168-177.

Drug Abuse Warning Network Report (2004), Amphetamine and methamphetamine emergency department visits, 1995-2002. *The DAWN Report*, July.

Derlet, R.W., Rice, P., Horowitz, B.Z. & Lord, R.V. (1989), Amphetamine toxicity: experience with 127 cases. *J. Emergency Medicine*, 7(2):157-61.

D'Onofrio, G. & Degutis, L.C. (2002), Preventive care in the emergency department: Screening and brief intervention for alcohol problems in the emergency department: A systematic review. *Academic Emergency Medicine*, 9(6), 627-638.

Hales, G., Roth, N. & Smith, D. (2000), Possible fatal interaction between protease inhibitors and methamphetamine. *Antiviral Therapy*, 5(1):19.

Harrington, R.D., Woodward, J.A., Hooton, T.M. & Horn, J.R. (1999), Life-threatening interactions between HIV-1 protease inhibitors and the illicit drugs MDMA and [gamma]-hydroxybutyrate. *Archives Internal Medicine*, 159(18):2221-2224.

Henry, J. (2001), Amphetamines. In: *Clinical Toxicology*, eds. M. Ford, K.A. Delaney, L. Ling & T. Erickson. Philadelphia: WB Saunders, pp. 620-626.

James, J.S. (2003), Antibiotic-resistant skin infections spreading among gay men, also in prisons. *AIDS Treatment News*, (388):2-3, Feb 7.

Jones, A.L. & Simpson, K.J. (1999), Mechanisms and management of hepatotoxicity in ecstasy (MDMA) and amphetamine intoxications. *Alimentary Pharmacology & Therapeutics*, 12:129-133.

Kalant, H., & Kalant, O.J. (1975), Death in amphetamine users: Causes and rates. *Canadian Medical J.*, 112:299-304.

Kamijo, Y., Soma, K., Nishida, M., Namera, A. & Ohwada, T. (2002), Acute liver failure following intravenous methamphetamine. *Veterinary & Human Toxicology*, 44(4):216-217.

Mohlesi, B. & Corbridge, T. (2003), Toxicology in the critically ill patient. *Clinics in Chest Medicine*, 24(4):689-711.

Moran, G.J. (2000), Pharmacologic management of HIV/STD exposure. *Emergency Medicine Clinics North America*, 18(4):829-842.

National Institute on Alcohol Abuse and Alcoholism (1995), *The Physician's Guide to Helping Patients with Alcohol Problems*. Washington, DC: Government Printing Office (NIH publication no. 95-3769).

Perez, J.A. Jr., Arsura, E.L. & Strategos, S. (1999), Methamphetamine-related stroke: Four cases. *J. Emergency Medicine*, 17(3):469-471.

Richards, J.R., Bretz, S.W., Johnson, E.B., Turnipseed, S.D., Brofeldt, B.T. & Derlet, R.W. (1999), Methamphetamine abuse and emergency department utilization. *Western J. Medicine*, 170(4):198-202.

Richards, J.R., Derlet, R.W. & Duncan, D.R. (1998), Chemical restraint for the agitated patient in the emergency department: Lorazepam versus droperidol. *J. Emergency Medicine*, 16(4):567-573.

Richards, J.R., Johnson, E.B., Stark, R.W. & Derlet, R.W. (1999), Methamphetamine abuse and rhabdomyolysis in the ED: A 5-year study. *American J. Emergency Medicine*, 17(7):681-685.

Rothrock, J.F., Rubenstein. R. & Lyden, P. (1988), Ischemic stroke associated with methamphetamine inhalation. *Neurology*, 38:589-592.

Rumbaugh, C.L., Bergeron, R.T., Scanlan, R.L., Teal, J.S., Segall, H.D., Fang, H.C. & McCormick, R. (1971), Cerebral vascular changes secondary to amphetamine abuse in the experimental animal. *Radiology*, 101:345-351.

Rumbaugh, C.L., Fang, H.C., Higgins, R.E., Bergeron, R.T., Segall, H.D. & Teal, J.S. (1976), Cerebral microvascular injury in experimental drug abuse. *Investigative Radiology*, 11(4):282-294.

Turnipseed, S.D., Richards, J.R., Kirk, J.D., Diercks, D.B. & Amsterdam, E.A. (2003), Frequency of acute coronary syndrome in patients presenting to the emergency department with chest pain after methamphetamine use. *J. Emergency Medicine*, 24(4):369-73.

Urbina, A. & Jones, K. (2004), Crystal Methamphetamine, its analogues, and HIV infection: Medical and psychiatric aspects of a new epidemic. *Clinical Infectious Diseases*, 38(6):890-894.

Varner, K.J., Ogden, B.A., Delcarpio, J. & Meleg-Smith, S. (2002), Cardiovascular responses elicited by the "binge" administration of methamphetamine. *J. Pharmacology & Experimental Therapeutics*, 301(1);152-159.

Wolff A.J. & O'Donnell, A.E. (2004), Pulmonary effects of illicit drug use. *Clinics in Chest Medicine*, 25(1):203-216.

APPENDIX

Referral Resources in New York City Metropolitan Area

1-800-Life-Net: NYC's 24 hour referral hotline for mental health and substance use treatment.

Callen-Lorde Community Health Center: 356 West 18th Street in Manhattan. (212) 271-7200. www.callen-lorde.org

Crystal Meth Anonymous: (212) 642-5029. www.nycma.org

Lesbian Gay Bisexual Transgender Community Center: 208 West 13th Street in Manhattan. (212) 620-7310. www.gaycenter.org

Gay Men's Health Crisis: 119 West 24th Street in Manhattan. (212) 376-1000. www.gmhc.org

Project PnP–Collaboration Between Chest (Center for HIV/AIDS Educational Studies and Training), Mount Sinai School of Medicine, Columbia University and Hunter University: (212) 206-7909 x 301.

Psychiatric Consequences
of Methamphetamine Use

Andrew J. Kolodny, MD

SUMMARY. Methamphetamine dependent individuals frequently suffer from co-occurring psychiatric disorders. These disorders may precede a methamphetamine use disorder or may result from methamphetamine use. Addressing co-occurring psychiatric disorders will improve methamphetamine treatment outcomes. Although effective pharmacological treatments for methamphetamine dependence are not yet available, psychiatric medications for anxiety and mood disorders are often needed. Methamphetamine dependence is treated with cognitive behavioral therapeutic approaches. *[Article copies available for a fee from The Haworth Document Delivery Service: 1-800-HAWORTH. E-mail address: <docdelivery@haworthpress.com> Website: <http://www.HaworthPress.com> © 2006 by The Haworth Press, Inc. All rights reserved.]*

KEYWORDS. Anxiety, cognitive behavioral therapy, co-occurring disorders, crystal meth, depression, dopamine, methamphetamine, motivational interviewing, psychosis, relapse prevention, stimulants

Andrew J. Kolodny is Medical Director–Special Projects, New York City Department of Health and Mental Hygiene.

Address correspondence to: Andrew J. Kolodny, MD, Office of the Executive Deputy Commissioner, NYC Department of Health & Mental Hygiene, 93 Worth Street, Room 1203, New York, NY 10013 (E-mail: Akolodny@health.nyc.gov).

[Haworth co-indexing entry note]: "Psychiatric Consequences of Methamphetamine Use." Kolodny, Andrew J. Co-published simultaneously in *Journal of Gay & Lesbian Psychotherapy* (The Haworth Medical Press, an imprint of The Haworth Press, Inc.) Vol. 10, No. 3/4, 2006, pp. 67-72; and: *Crystal Meth and Men Who Have Sex with Men: What Mental Health Care Professionals Need to Know* (ed: Milton L. Wainberg, Andrew J. Kolodny, and Jack Drescher) The Haworth Medical Press, an imprint of The Haworth Press, Inc., 2006, pp. 67-72. Single or multiple copies of this article are available for a fee from The Haworth Document Delivery Service [1-800-HAWORTH, 9:00 a.m. - 5:00 p.m. (EST). E-mail address: docdelivery@haworthpress.com].

Methamphetamine is a highly addictive stimulant. It can be snorted, smoked, taken orally, intravenously, or anally. Methamphetamine use results in short-term feelings of euphoria and increased motor activity. Heavy or prolonged methamphetamine use can cause long-lasting damage to brain neurons (Ernst et al., 2000).

To better understand methamphetamine's mechanism of action and how its use can rapidly progress to addiction, it is helpful to review how the limbic system (the brain's reward circuitry) functions in the natural state. When one engages in a naturally pleasurable activity, such as eating or having sex, the neurotransmitter dopamine is released causing activation of the limbic center. This activation leads to a feeling of satisfaction and pleasure that serves as a positive reinforcement.

Methamphetamine and cocaine have a similar mechanism of action. Both of these drugs act by causing massive amounts of dopamine to enter the space between neurons, thus leading to over-stimulation of the limbic system. Unlike cocaine, which exerts its effects on the external cell membrane, methamphetamine has a much longer duration of action and acts inside the cell. Methamphetamine produces its effects by interfering with normal intracellular processes (Pifl et al., 2000). The longer duration of action and the fact that it acts intracellularly, may explain why methamphetamine appears to be far more toxic to brain neurons than cocaine.

From an evolutionary standpoint, one can easily appreciate how positively reinforced behaviors, such as eating or having sex, are important for survival and for passing one's genes to the next generation. However, artificially activating this system with methamphetamine can significantly impair normal psychological and cognitive functioning.

METHAMPHETAMINE INTOXICATION

Pleasant symptoms of acute methamphetamine intoxication include feelings of euphoria, satisfaction, and a sense of well-being. Unpleasant effects include restlessness, irritability, insomnia and loss of appetite. Aggressive and violent behavior during acute intoxication may also occur.

Methamphetamine intoxication can mimic a variety of psychiatric problems, including mood disorders, psychotic disorders, and anxiety disorders. Flight of ideas, euphoria, grandiosity, irritability, mood liability, impulsivity, and hyper-sexuality are symptoms that define a manic episode but are also commonly experienced during methamphetamine intoxication.

Psychotic symptoms are more likely to occur in the context of heavy or prolonged methamphetamine use. These symptoms can include paranoid delusions as well as auditory hallucinations (Kunio et al., 2000). When these symptoms develop, immediate psychiatric attention, antipsychotic medication, and close monitoring may be indicated. Psychotic symptoms are usually time-limited and resolve when methamphetamine use is discontinued, but may reoccur with further use.

Symptoms resembling anxiety disorders often occur during methamphetamine intoxication. Panic attacks and agoraphobia in the context of methamphetamine use have been reported (Iwanami et al., 1997). Symptoms of a panic attack that methamphetamine users may experience include intense fear, diaphoresis (profuse sweating), palpitations, and a sense of losing control or impending doom.

Compulsive behaviors can occur and include activities such as excessive cleaning or engaging in compulsive sexual behavior. The latter is particularly concerning because of its association with an increase in sexual risk behaviors for the transmission of HIV or other sexually transmitted infections. Repetitive, stereotypical motor behaviors, known as "punding," arise during intoxication with methamphetamine (Schiorring, 1981). Punding behaviors include repetitive handling and examining of one's own body part or foreign objects, such as picking at oneself or taking apart mechanical devices. Repetitive sorting and arranging of one's belongings are also seen.

METHAMPHETAMINE WITHDRAWAL

About 8 hours after using methamphetamine, there is typically a sharp decline in mood and energy levels. This period may last for days and can be associated with an intense craving to use again. Unlike withdrawal from alcohol or sedatives, methamphetamine withdrawal generally does not lead to life threatening physical complications. However, severe depressive symptoms associated with suicidal ideation may occur and require emergency psychiatric intervention.

The symptoms of methamphetamine withdrawal closely resemble a major depressive episode. Symptoms such as depressed mood, anhedonia, psychomotor retardation, fatigue, sleep disturbance (hypersomnia or insomnia) are seen in both conditions. The clinician should try to determine if depressive symptoms preceded methamphetamine use. In reality, it is often very difficult to clearly distinguish a pre-existing depressive disorder from a methamphetamine induced depressive disorder. If the individual used small quantities of methamphetamine for a brief duration, methamphetamine induced depressive symptoms should improve quickly and may not require antidepressant medication.

Following heavy or protracted methamphetamine use, mood and anxiety symptoms as well as cognitive difficulties may persist for several weeks or longer. Recent brain imaging studies have demonstrated that methamphetamine causes long-lasting damage to the brain in areas associated with depressive and anxiety disorders (London et al., 2004). Psychiatric medication may help alleviate these symptoms.

CO-OCCURRING PSYCHIATRIC DISORDERS

The possibility of a pre-existing or substance-induced mood or anxiety disorder should be considered in every patient that presents for treatment of methamphetamine addiction. Treatment for co-occurring psychiatric conditions will contribute to more effective addiction treatment. In addition to psychotherapy, pharmacological interventions to target co-occurring psychiatric disorders are often required. Diagnoses that should be considered include the following:

- Polysubstance Abuse and Dependence
- Major Depressive Disorder
- Bipolar Disorder
- Anxiety Disorders
- Post Traumatic Stress Disorder
- Personality Disorders

Patients who present for treatment of addiction to methamphetamine should be screened for these disorders. If a co-occurring mental illness is suspected, patients should be referred for psychiatric evaluation as quickly as possible. Treating mood and anxiety disorders in these patients enables them to cope better with recovery.

TREATMENT OF METHAMPHETAMINE ADDICTION

Pharmacological treatments for stimulant dependence are not yet available. Effective treatment options primarily consist of psychosocial interventions. These techniques include the following:

Community Reinforcement is an approach that promotes recovery oriented lifestyle changes. This individualized form of treatment addresses key areas such as relationships, employment, social networks, and recreational practices (Smith, Meyers and Miller, 2001).

Contingency Management is a technique that can decrease drug use by providing an immediate reward to an individual for remaining drug free. Voucher-based incentives are a type of contingency management approach that reward an individual for a negative urine toxicology result with a voucher that can be exchanged for retail items (Higgins, Alessi and Dantona, 2002).

Relapse Prevention is an approach that teaches patients new skills to cope with craving as well as strategies to prevent a relapse should an individual have a slip. Patients also learn how to avoid placing themselves in situations that might lead to relapse (Brown et al., 2002).

Couples Therapy brings an individual's significant other into the treatment setting. Including significant others in treatment can improve outcomes by improving the stability of the patient's relationships (Rawson, 1999).

The Matrix Model is a manualized model that integrates a variety of psychosocial treatment approaches such as relapse prevention, motivational interviewing, urine toxicology testing. Treatment is delivered over a defined period of time and consists of individual and group sessions as well as encouragement of 12 step program involvement (Rawson et al., 1995).

Psychiatric consequences of methamphetamine use as well as pre-existing mental illnesses in the methamphetamine user must be addressed. Treatment settings that are able to offer integrated addiction and mental health treatment are likely to retain patients longer and achieve better treatment outcomes.

REFERENCES

Brown, T.G., Seraganian, P., Tremblay, J. & Annis, H. (2002), Process and outcome changes with relapse prevention versus 12-Step aftercare programs for substance abusers. *Addiction*, 97(6):677-89.

Ernst, T., Chang, L., Leonido-Yee, M. & Speck, O. (2000), Evidence for long-term neurotoxicity associated with methamphetamine abuse. *Neurology*, 54:1344-1349.

Iwanami, A., Kuwakado, D., Otsubo, T., Ishono, H. & Kamijima, K. (1997), Relapse of panic disorder induced by a single intravenous methamphetamine injection. *J Anxiety Disorders*, 11(1):113-116.

London, E.D., Simon, S.L., Berman, S.M., Mandelkern, M.A., Lichtman, A.M., Bramen, J., Shinn, A.K., Miotto, K., Learn, J., Dong, Y., Matochik, J.A., Kurian, V., Newton, T., Woods, R., Rawson, R. & Ling, W. (2004), Mood disturbances and regional cerebral metabolic abnormalities in recently abstinent methamphetamine abusers. *Archives General Psychiatry*, 61(1):73-84.

Pifl, C., Sitte, H.H., Reither, H. & Singer, E.A. (2000), The mechanism of the releasing action of amphetamine. Uptake, superfusion, and electrophysiological studies on transporter-transfected cells. *Pure Applied Chemistry*, 72:1045-1050.

Rawson, R.A. (1999), *Treatment of Stimulant Use Disorders (Treatment Improvement Protocol (TIP) #33)*. Rockville, MD: US Department of Health & Human Services.

Rawson, R.A., Shoptaw, S.J., Obert, J.L., McCann, M.J., Hasson, A.L., Marinelli-Casey, P.J., Brethen, P.R. & Ling, W. (1995), An intensive outpatient approach for cocaine abuse treatment: The Matrix model. *J Substance Abuse Treatment*, 12(2): 117-127.

Schiorring, E. (1981), Psychopathology induced by "speed drugs." *Pharmacology Biochemistry & Behavior*, 14(Suppl 1):109-122.

Smith, J.E., Meyers, R.J. & Miller, W.R. (2001), The community reinforcement approach to the treatment of substance use disorders. *American J Addictions*, 10(Suppl): 51-9.

Yui, K., Ikemoto, S., Ishiguro, T. & Goto, K. (2000), Studies of amphetamine or methamphetamine psychosis in Japan: Relation of methamphetamine psychosis to schizophrenia. *Annals New York Academy of Sciences*, 914:1-12.

Crystal Methamphetamine
Use and Sexually Transmitted Infection:
The Importance of Sexual History Taking

Susan Blank, MD, MPH

SUMMARY. Crystal methamphetamine (MA) use is associated with sexual behaviors that increase the risk of HIV and other sexually transmitted infections (STIs). Sexual history-taking and screening for sexually transmitted infections can be a powerful way for primary care clinicians to identify and address crystal meth and other substance abuse problems. The reverse is also true: patients with known substance abuse or mental health problems may benefit greatly from careful sexual health evaluation and counseling. As the majority of STIs have no noticeable symptoms in their early stages, clinicians diagnosing crystal methamphetamine or other substance abuse problems, or taking care of the primary care needs of such patients must be familiar with sexual history-taking in order to identify patients needing a thorough exam and to ensure adequate STI screening. *[Article copies available for a fee from The Haworth Document Delivery Service: 1-800-HAWORTH. E-mail address: <docdelivery@haworthpress.com> Website: <http://www.HaworthPress.com> © 2006 by The Haworth Press, Inc. All rights reserved.]*

Susan Blank is affiliated with the New York City Department of Health and Mental Hygiene, Bureau of Sexually Transmitted Disease Control, New York City, NY, USA; and the Division of STD Prevention, National Center for HIV, STD, and TB Prevention, Centers for Disease Control and Prevention, Atlanta, GA, USA.

Address correspondence to: Susan Blank, MD, MPH, New York City Department of Health and Mental Hygiene, Bureau of Sexually Transmitted Disease Control, 125 Worth Street, CN #73, New York, NY 10013 (E-mail: sblank@health.nyc.gov).

[Haworth co-indexing entry note]: "Crystal Methamphetamine Use and Sexually Transmitted Infection: The Importance of Sexual History Taking." Blank, Susan. Co-published simultaneously in *Journal of Gay & Lesbian Psychotherapy* (The Haworth Medical Press, an imprint of The Haworth Press, Inc.) Vol. 10, No. 3/4, 2006, pp. 73-84; and: *Crystal Meth and Men Who Have Sex with Men: What Mental Health Care Professionals Need to Know* (ed: Milton L. Wainberg, Andrew J. Kolodny, and Jack Drescher) The Haworth Medical Press, an imprint of The Haworth Press, Inc., 2006, pp. 73-84. Single or multiple copies of this article are available for a fee from The Haworth Document Delivery Service [1-800-HAWORTH, 9:00 a.m. - 5:00 p.m. (EST). E-mail address: docdelivery@haworthpress.com].

KEYWORDS. Chlamydia, crystal meth, gonorrhea, herpes, homosexuality, methamphetamine, men who have sex with men (MSM), sexual history, sexually transmitted infection (STI)

In the U.S. each year, there are an estimated 15 million new cases of sexually transmitted infections (STIs) (Figure 1). Though much more frequently occurring than HIV, STIs such as human papilloma virus, trichomonas, chlamydia, herpes and gonorrhea receive considerably less media and public attention despite their significant burden of morbidity. Most STIs have no presenting symptoms and may not prompt a person to seek care. It is a minority of STIs that present with recognizable symptoms, such as genital ulcers, genital discharge, rashes or growths.

Left untreated, STIs can result in pelvic inflammatory disease, chronic pelvic pain, ectopic pregnancy, and infertility (due to chlamydia, gonorrhea), cancers (cervical and anal cancer due to human papilloma virus; hepatocellular cancer due to hepatitis), adverse outcomes of pregnancy

FIGURE 1. Estimated Number of New STD Cases per Year, U.S.

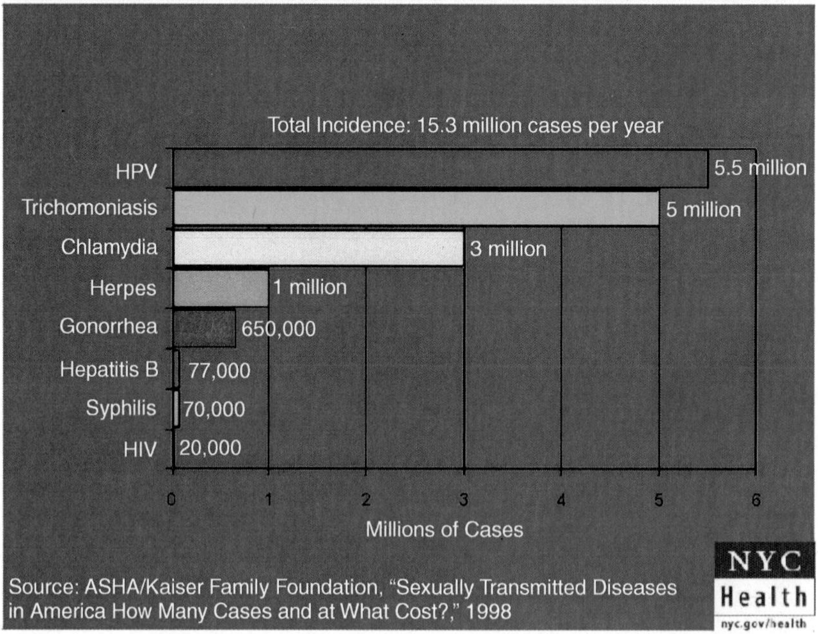

Total Incidence: 15.3 million cases per year

	Millions of Cases
HPV	5.5 million
Trichomoniasis	5 million
Chlamydia	3 million
Herpes	1 million
Gonorrhea	650,000
Hepatitis B	77,000
Syphilis	70,000
HIV	20,000

Source: ASHA/Kaiser Family Foundation, "Sexually Transmitted Diseases in America How Many Cases and at What Cost?," 1998

NYC
Health
nyc.gcv/health

(stillbirth due to syphilis, prematurity due to trichomonas; invasive eye infection due to gonorrhea and lung disease of the newborn due to chlamydia). Moreover, HIV behaves synergistically with other STIs (Eng and Butler, 1997). The presence of one facilitates the transmission of another. This is especially true for ulcerative STIs, which interrupt the body's most important first line of defense–intact skin and mucous membranes. Conversely, if an HIV-uninfected person has an STI other than HIV, the cells that HIV infects are recruited to the site of infection, so that they become easier targets for the virus that causes HIV (Fleming and Wasserheit, 1999).

Sexual risk assessments are frequently inadequate. To measure the adequacy of patient histories, in general, the Kaiser Family Foundation interviewed women across the US who had just completed a first patient visit with an obstetrician-gynecologist. Approximately 74% of women reported that the physician discussed breast self-examination and/or Pap smear, but only 39% reported that the physician discussed sexual history (Hoff and James, 1997). This statistic is especially notable, as obstetrics and gynecology is a medical subspecialty devoted to reproductive health issues. Other clinicians may be less attuned to sexual health by virtue of a lack of clinical training in this area, clinician discomfort, concern about offending patients with such questions, and time constraints.

There are also many missed opportunities for STI screening and treatment. Chlamydia in women is a prime example. Uncomplicated chlamydia is generally clinically "silent," and if untreated can lead to facilitated HIV transmission, chronic pelvic pain, ectopic pregnancy, infertility or adverse pregnancy outcomes. Uncomplicated infection is readily treated with a single dose of antibiotic (Centers for Disease Control (CDC), 2002). In 2002, of the 654,464 cases of chlamydia reported in the United States, 76% occurred among women 15-24 years (CDC, 2003a). Recognizing the importance of chlamydia, the US Preventive Health Services Task Force (1996) recommends chlamydia screening for all sexually active women under the age of 26 years. This recommendation was adopted by the National Committee for Quality Assurance (NCQA), the leading accrediting agency for managed care organizations, as one of its "report card" measures for managed care plans. These "report cards" provide purchasers of health insurance with information on such areas as patient satisfaction, delivery of preventive services, and cost (CDC, 2004b).

In the United States, screening rates for sexually active females 16-26 years in 2001 were 26% in commercial plans and 38% in Medicaid plans (CDC, 2004b). In New York State in 2003, the State Department of

Health's Office of Managed Care reported that approximately 30% of sexually active women 16-26 years old enrolled in commercial managed care plans had an annual Chlamydia screening test, and approximately 38% of sexually active women 16-26 years old enrolled in Medicaid managed care plans were screened (New York State Department of Health, 2003). These data underscore gaps in the provision of sexual health care among primary care clinicians. Members of the psychiatric community can help patients by identifying triggers for STI screening, and developing a referral network for the STI screening of their patients (if screening cannot be done on-site).

BASICS OF SEXUAL HISTORY-TAKING

In taking a sexual history, it is important to set the stage for open and ongoing, non-judgmental dialogue (Blank, 1993; also see Table 1). For minors, this may include introducing parents to the privacy needs of their children. As an introductory statement, a clinician can state, "In order to give you the best care possible, there are some things I need to know about you. For example, what you are eating; what your exercise habits are; how much alcohol you drink and how often; your use of non-prescription drugs and street drugs, your sexual practices and how you think life is going for you. Please jump in with anything you want to speak with me about, especially if I didn't ask."

Clinicians need to be careful to avoid assumptions and unwarranted interpretations of a patient's meaning. This means clinicians should not assume that:

- sex means only anal or vaginal intercourse
- oral sex is "safe"
- well-dressed patients have no drug or domestic violence problems
- married people are monogamous
- pregnant women have only 1 sex partner, or the same partner throughout a pregnancy
- persons who self-identity as heterosexual have no same-sex partners
- persons identifying themselves as gay or lesbian have no opposite sex partners
- older people don't have sex

To get at the information needed for the exam, the clinician should ask such specifics as: when was the last date of sexual exposure; the number

TABLE 1. Sexual History Basics

- Set the stage for open, ongoing, non-judgmental discussion
- Make no assumptions: such short cuts may lead you down the wrong path
- Tailor your language in order to obtain the right information
  - Ask about actual sexual behaviors – what orifices, how often, barrier protection, how many different sex partners over the interval of interest; and STI symptoms
  - Explore patient's psychosocial history, including drug use, mental health, and history of physical or sexual abuse
- Make the most of counseling opportunities

and nature of different sexual partners over the last 6 months–and specifically the number of male partners and the number of female partners; and steady versus casual or anonymous partners. It is also important to understand which sites were exposed–oral, vaginal or anal cavities or other sites, and whether the patient has been an insertive or receptive partner, or both–to help focus the exam and appropriate specimen collection. It is also important to inquire about the use of barriers, such as condoms, with *each* type of sexual behavior. For example, a patient who engages in oral and vaginal sex may report using a condom every time. On closer questioning, the patient acknowledges that condoms were used only during vaginal or anal sex, but not with oral sex–and the patient does not ever use condoms for oral sex. This is not an insignificant omission insofar as oral sex is a possible mode of transmission for STIs, especially in the presence of oral micro-trauma and abrasions.

In addition to sexual behavior, clinicians should assess the psychosocial milieu. This is done by asking questions about depression, anxiety, self-esteem, alcohol and drug use in general, especially substance use before and during sex, recent travel and new sex/needle partners while traveling, age at first sexual activity, history of physical or sexual abuse, current contraceptive needs, past STI history–including HIV testing history, and any current STI symptoms–such as genital ulcers, discharges, rashes or rectal pain.

For example, one of the effects of crystal methamphetamine is increased libido. In men, that libido can exceed the ability to have and maintain erections throughout the course of a several-day binge of sexual activity. Men under the influence of crystal methamphetamine have reported engaging in sexual behaviors unlikely to occur in the absence of that drug use. They may cease to use barrier protection or may engage in receptive anal intercourse when they might not otherwise. It is not surprising, then, that there has been increasing evidence associating crystal methamphetamine use with STI (Paz-Bailey et al., 2004; Mitchell et al., 2004; Mansergh et al., 2004; Urbina and Jones, 2004).

The sexual behavior history and any symptom history can help guide the examination. Risky sexual behaviors warranting further assessment include: more than a single mutually monogamous sex partner during the last 6 months (or history interval)–whether with concurrent or serial partners;[1] unprotected sex outside a mutually monogamous relationship; any involvement in bartering money or drugs for sex, or vice versa, use of alcohol and other drugs recreationally; a history of recent STI or documented STI in a current sex partner.

THE STI-FOCUSED PHYSICAL EXAM

The STI-focused exam includes inspection of all skin surfaces, including genital and anal, the scalp, the palms of the hands and the soles of the feet, as one can detect evidence of herpes, genital warts, and syphilitic rashes in these areas. Oral examination may reveal not only evidence of crystal meth abuse, but also evidence of HIV (thrush, oral hairy leukoplakia), syphilis (primary chancre or mucous patches) or gonorrhea (pharyngitis). Lymph node palpation (cervical, clavicular, axillary, epitrochlear, inguinal) may reveal enlargement in the presence of HIV, syphilis, chancroid, lymphogranuloma venereum and herpes. Inspection of the external genitalia, the perineum, and anus may reveal herpetic, syphilitic or other ulcers, genital warts, other growths, or discharge. Close exam of the male urethra can yield clues to urethritis, and the pelvic exam can yield clues to cervicitis, pelvic inflammatory disease, and vaginitis. Also, patients engaging in anal receptive intercourse should have a careful anal assessment.

SCREENING, LABORATORY ASSESSMENT AND TREATMENT

Basic STI screening tests are summarized in Table 2 and screening recommendations for special populations in Table 3.

Any of the following behaviors should trigger STI screening by laboratory testing (Blank, 1993):

- Sex without a condom–especially anal intercourse
- Sex with more than one partner

- Sex with injection drug users or prostitutes
- Sex with a partner who is infected with HIV or another STI.

Additionally, sexual behavior may be determined within the milieu of a variety of psychosocial factors. This includes exploration of psychosocial issues that can influence sexual risk-taking (such as substance abuse, mental illness, child sexual abuse and partner violence), as well as specifics of sexual risk taking.

For patients with histories that place them at risk for STI, laboratory screening for epidemiologically relevant STIs (including HIV) should be performed. For patients sexually exposed to an individual(s) known to be infected, or those with recognizable symptoms of infection, collect the necessary laboratory specimens, and treat presumptively. Waiting for results delays treatment, risks patient loss to follow up and the development of serious long-term sequelae in the patient, and spread of infection to partners. Because many STIs are spread via the same sexual behaviors,

TABLE 2. STI Screening Basics: Recommend Tests and Collection Sites

Pathogen	Test Types	Site of Specimen Collection
Chlamydia/gonorrhea	Culture;* DNA probe; Nucleic acid amplification tests	Oral/Anal;* Urethral/ Cervical swab Urine[†] Vaginal swab
Hepatitis B	Serology	Blood
Syphilis (Treponema pallidum)	Serology	Blood
HIV	Serology	Blood; Oral fluid
HPV-related cancers	Pap test	Cervix; anus[‡]
Trichomonas	Culture; Saline microscopy, culture, Antigen detection test	Vaginal fluid/urethral swab

* Culture is the only FDA cleared test for the oropharynx, or the anus (e.g., for men or women engaging in oral and/or anal sex). Also, chlamydia or gonorrhea culture is the only test for the work up of child sexual abuse which is admissible in a court of law.

[†] Urine testing is available only via nucleic acid amplification techniques.

[‡] Some practitioners advocate anal pap smears for men who have sex with men and some for women engaging in anal sex (especially among men and women who are HIV-infected), although this practice is not currently recommended by the Centers for Disease Control and Prevention.

N.B. Routine serologic screening for Herpes Simplex Virus is not currently recommended by CDC.

TABLE 3. STI screening and vaccine recommendations for special populations

HIV+ Persons [0] MMWR (CDC, 2003b)	Men who have sex with men MMWR (CDC, 2002)	Pregnant Women MMWR (CDC, 2002)
	HIV test	HIV test
Urogential Chlamydia [6] Urogenital Gonorrhea	Urogential Chlamydia Urogenital Gonorrhea	Urogential Chlamydia Urogenital Gonorrhea
Rectal Chlamydia [1] Rectal Gonorrhea [1]	Rectal Chlamydia [1] Rectal Gonorrhea [1	
Oral Gonorrhea [2]	Oral Gonorrhea [2]	
Syphilis serology	Syphilis serology	Syphilis serology
Herpes type-specific serology [3a]	Herpes type-specific serology [3b]	
Hepatitis B vaccine, if susceptible Hepatitis A vaccine, if susceptible	Hepatitis B vaccine, if susceptible Hepatitis A vaccine, if susceptible	Hepatitis B surface Ag
Cervical Cancer screen [4]		Cervical Cancer screen
Vaginal Trichomonas (women)		
Bacterail vaginosis (women) [3]		Bacterial vaginosis [5]
Anal Pap Test†	Anal Pap Test†	

[0] Baseline screening activities. Repeat at least annually if interim patient history reveals ongoing risks, such as:
- Multiple or anonymous partners
- History of previous STI
- Identification of psychosocial behaviors associated with the spread of HIV or other STD, such as crystal methamphetamine use, use of poppers, depression, low self esteem
- Developmental or lifetime changes that may lead to increased risk-taking (e.g., dissoluation of a relationship)
- Partners with any of these risks

[1] If patient has history of receptive anal intercourse
[2] If patient has history of receptive oral sex
[3a] Not recommended by the Centers for Disease Control and Prevention; recommended by California STD Controllers Association and California Coalition of Local Aids Directors (2001)
[3b] Not recommended by the Centers for Disease Control and Prevention; recommended by Public Health Seattle and King County (2001)
[4] Women only. Twice during the first year after HIV diagnosis, and if normal, annually thereafter.
[5] If at risk of pre-term labor
[6] If <= 25 years or if at increased risk of STI–see [0]

† Some experts advocate anal Pap test for HIV-infected persons engaging in anal sex, although this practice is not currently recommended by the Centers for Disease Control and Prevention.

sample collection should include testing for other STIs as well, including HIV if current HIV status is unknown.[2]

Treatment regimens are clearly articulated by the Centers for Disease Control and Prevention, in the latest CDC STD Treatment Guidelines.[3] Updates are published as needed in the CDC's weekly publication, the Morbidity and Mortality Weekly Report (MMWR) (CDC, 2004a). In general, the recommended regimens for uncomplicated and curable STI (chlamydia, gonorrhea, trichomonas, and primary, secondary and early latent syphilis) are single dose options which can be taken under the direct observation of the clinician. By not necessitating multiple doses, single dose therapy does not rely on the patient remembering to take doses, and does not require medication storage by the patient, which is important for persons who might otherwise need to store or even conceal a full course of medications (e.g., adolescents, homeless persons, and persons in socially chaotic situations).

In the short term, patients requiring STI treatment should be advised at the time of treatment to avoid sex until all medications are completed, any existing symptoms are gone and all current sex partners have been evaluated and/or treated.

Ideally, infected persons will notify all of their at-risk partners. This may not always be possible-patients may be willing to inform certain partners, but not others. Clinicians can play an important role in notifying partners and facilitating their treatment. First, explain the importance of treating partners to avoid patient re-infection or spread of infection to others. Next, explore the patient's comfort in notifying partners and his/her plan for doing so. The patient may need guidance in what and how to tell a partner directly; the patient may require the presence of a third party in order to tell a partner; or the patient may want to have the partner notified, but may not want to participate in the notification process. It should also be expected that some patients will not want to either discuss partners or wish to have partners notified. Participation in the partner notification process is voluntary on the part of the patient, but state law may have provision for the clinician or public health authority to notify any known partners, including spouses, depending on the situation.

Clinicians choosing to notify partners on behalf of the patient should never reveal the identity of the patient to the partner. Alternatively, the state or local health department may be able to provide assistance to the patient and/or clinician upon request. The clinician is not legally obligated to evaluate partners. However, if partners require assistance accessing care, the index patient should be educated regarding relevant confidentiality laws and safety net providers (e.g., local health department or public hospital services), in case partners need them. If timely evaluation and treatment is in doubt, in some states, providers can give index patients medication (or prescriptions) for partners (Klausner and Chaw, 2003).

SEXUAL BEHAVIOR COUNSELING

In addition to identifying who needs screening, and whether or not a STI diagnosis is made, the sexual risk assessment may also identify important areas for counseling and prevention activities. A patient's self-perceived risk may need to be reconciled with the actual risk. Clinicians may need to help the patient recognize barriers to STI risk reduction and support achievable patient STI risk reduction strategies. Critical strategies include reducing the number of sex partners, carrying condoms in all situations where sexual activity may occur, and ensuring that patients know how to get the best protection from condoms. Importantly, sexual risk assessment may help identify other coexisting conditions requiring attention (e.g., substance abuse, depression, or sexual abuse)–especially as these conditions may interact and amplify each other (Stall et al., 2003).

Over the course of a longitudinal clinician-patient relationship, changes in behaviors over time should be examined–either to reinforce positive changes or identify and address emergent or persistent risky behaviors (i.e., not just negative changes but the lack of change at all). Similarly, if any of these co-existing conditions (e.g., substance abuse, mental illness, history of physical or sexual abuse) are previously known to the clinician, an understanding of these conditions can help focus the sexual risk assessment. Crystal methamphetamine abuse, for example, can influence partner selection, behaviors with each partner, and attention to prevention. Thus, the clinician should work with the patient to prevent secondary sequelae while addressing the primary problem. Lastly, the patient's sexual history can identify primary prevention opportunities, such as ensuring immunization for hepatitis B and hepatitis A–the only vaccine-preventable STIs–as appropriate.

CONCLUSION

Sexual histories help identify patients in need of STI screening–and thus are key to preventing the spread and sequelae of STI. The presence of psychosocial factors which can influence sexual behavior underscores the need for concomitant sexual history-taking and STI screening. Similarly, sexual histories may help uncover other serious health and behavioral problems.

NOTES

1. Concurrent partners pose greater risk for rapid spread of infection; however, it is not uncommon–especially for adolescents–to have multiple, serial partners in rapid succession, but one at a time, and to consider themselves monogamous, and thus at low STI risk.
2. Some manufacturers simplify this by making possible dual testing, e.g., for chlamydia and gonorrhea using a single specimen.
3. These are re-issued by CDC every 3-5 years; most recently, in 2002.

REFERENCES

Blank, S. (1993), STDs: Are you looking for them? Do you know what to do when you find them? *City Health Information*, 12(3):1-4.

California STD Controllers Association and California coalition of Local Aids Directors (2001), Guidance for STD clinical preventive services for persons infected with HIV. *Sexually Transmitted Diseases*, 28(8):460-463.

Centers for Disease Control & Prevention (2002), Sexually transmitted diseases treatment guidelines 2002. *Morbidity & Mortality Weekly Report*, 51 (No. RR-6):1-80. http://www.cdc.gov/ mmwr/PDF/RR/RR5106.pdf.

Centers for Disease Control & Prevention (2003a), *Sexually Transmitted Disease Surveillance, 2002*. Atlanta, GA: U.S. Department of Health and Human Services, September.

Centers for Disease Control & Prevention (2003b), Incorporating HIV prevention into the medical care of persons living with HIV: recommendations of the CDC, Health Resources Administration, the National Institutes of Health and the HIV Medicine Association of the Infectious Diseases Society of American, 2003. *Morbidity and Mortality Weekly Report*, 52(No. RR-12):1-24.

Centers for Disease Control & Prevention (2004a), Increases in fluoroquinolone-resistant neisseria gonorrhoeae among men who have sex with men–United States, 2003, and revised recommendations for gonorrhea treatment, 2004. *Morbidity & Mortality Weekly Report*, 53:335-338.

Centers for Disease Control & Prevention (2004b), Chlamydia screening among sexually active young females enrollees of health plans–United States, 1999-2001. *Morbidity & Mortality Weekly Report*, 53:983-985. *http://www.cdc.gov/mmwr/PDF/wk/mm5316.pdf*

Eng, T.R. & Butler, W.T. eds. (1997), *The Hidden Epidemic: Confronting Sexually Transmitted Diseases*. Washington, DC: National Academy Press.

Fleming, D.T. & Wasserheit, J.N. (1999), From epidemiological synergy to public health policy and practice: The contribution of other sexually transmitted diseases to sexual transmission of HIV infection. *Sexually Transmitted Infections*, 75(1): 3-17.

Hoff, T. & James, M. (1997), *Talking about STDs with Health Professionals: Women's Experiences*. Kaiser Family Foundation. Package #1313. September 17.

Klausner, J.D. & Chaw, J.K. (2003), Patient-delivered therapy for chlamydia: Putting research into practice. *Sexually Transmitted Diseases*, 30(6):509-511.

Mansergh, G., Shouse. R.L., Marks, G., Rader, M., Buchbinder, S. & Colfax, G.N. (2004), *Crystal Use, Viagra Use, and Specific Sexual Risk Behaviors of Men Who Have Sex with Men (MSM) During a Recent Anal Sex Encounter*. Abstract D04B, National STD Prevention Conference. Philadelphia, PA, March.

Mitchell, S.J., Wong, W., Kent, C.K., Chaw, J.K. & Klausner, J.D. (2004), *Methamphetamine Use, Sexual Behavior, and Sexually Transmitted Diseases Among Men Who Have Sex with Men Seen in an STD Clinic, San Francisco 2002-2003*. Abstract D04C, National STD Prevention Conference. Philadelphia, PA, March.

New York State Department of Health (2003), New York State Managed Care Plan Performance: A Report on Quality, Access to Care and Customer Satisfaction. http://www.health.state.ny.us/nysdoh/mancare/qarrfull/qarr_2003/qarr2003.pdf. Accessed November 5, 2004.

Paz-Bailey, G., Meyers, A., Blank, S., Brown, J., Rubin, S., Braxton, J., Zaidi, A., Schafzin, J., Weigl, S. & Markowitz, L. (2004), A case-control study of syphilis among men who have sex with men in New York City: Association with HIV infection. *Sexually Transmitted Diseases*, 31(10):581-587.

Public Health Seattle and King County (2001), Sexually transmitted Disease and HIV screening guidelines for men who have sex with men. *Sexually Transmitted Diseases*, 28(8):457-459.

Stall, R., Mills, T.C., Williamson, J., Hart, T., Greenwood, G., Paul, J., Pollack, L., Binson, D,. Osmond, D. & Catania, J.A. (2003), Association of co-occurring psychosocial health problems and increased vulnerability to HIV/AIDS among urban men who have sex with men. *American J. Public Health*, 93:939-942.

Urbina, A. & Jones, K. (2004), Crystal methamphetamine, its analogues and HIV infection: Medical and psychiatric aspects of a new epidemic. *Clinical Infections Diseases*, 38:890-894.

US Preventive Health Services Task Force (1996), *Guide to Clinical Preventive Services, 2nd ed*. Available at http://ww.ahrq.gov/clinic.cpsix/htm. Accessed November 5, 2004.

Crystal Methamphetamine Use Among Men Who Have Sex with Men: Results from Two National Online Studies

Sabina Hirshfield, PhD
Robert H. Remien, PhD
Mary Ann Chiasson, DrPH

SUMMARY. This paper describes crystal methamphetamine (crystal) use and sexual risk behaviors for two web-based surveys of men who have sex with men (MSM). The subjects were recruited online. Crystal

Sabina Hirshfield is Deputy Director of Research and Evaluation, and Mary Ann Chiasson is Vice President of Research and Evaluation, Medical and Health Research Association of New York City, Inc., New York, NY.

Robert H. Remien, is Associate Professor of Clinical Psychology, HIV Center for Clinical and Behavioral Studies, New York State Psychiatric Institute and Columbia University, New York, NY.

Address correspondence to: Sabina Hirshfield, PhD, Medical and Health Research Association of New York City, Inc., 22 Church Street, 5th Floor, New York, NY 10013 (E-mail: shirshfield@mhra.org).

This work was funded in part through CDC Contract Number 200-97-0621, Task 33 to RTI International, and Subcontract Number 10-46U-6900 from RTI to Medical and Health Research Association of New York City, Inc. The content of this publication does not necessarily reflect the views or policies of the Department of Health and Human Services, nor does mention of trade names, commercial products, or organizations imply endorsement by the U.S. Government.

[Haworth co-indexing entry note]: "Crystal Methamphetamine Use Among Men Who Have Sex with Men: Results from Two National Online Studies." Hirshfield, Sabina, Robert H. Remien, and Mary Ann Chiasson. Co-published simultaneously in *Journal of Gay & Lesbian Psychotherapy* (The Haworth Medical Press, an imprint of The Haworth Press, Inc.) Vol. 10, No. 3/4, 2006, pp. 85-93; and: *Crystal Meth and Men Who Have Sex with Men: What Mental Health Care Professionals Need to Know* (ed: Milton L. Wainberg, Andrew J. Kolodny, and Jack Drescher) The Haworth Medical Press, an imprint of The Haworth Press, Inc., 2006, pp. 85-93. Single or multiple copies of this article are available for a fee from The Haworth Document Delivery Service [1-800-HAWORTH, 9:00 a.m. - 5:00 p.m. (EST). E-mail address: docdelivery@haworthpress.com].

use was associated with young age, having a greater number of sex partners, having unprotected anal intercourse (UAI), having a sexually transmitted infection (STI), and being HIV-positive. Significant regional differences were seen in the prevalence of crystal use. Findings are discussed in relation to the need to integrate messages about the relationship between drug use and sexual behavior into HIV prevention programs. *[Article copies available for a fee from The Haworth Document Delivery Service: 1-800-HAWORTH. E-mail address: <docdelivery@haworthpress.com> Website: <http://www.HaworthPress.com> © 2006 by The Haworth Press, Inc. All rights reserved.]*

KEYWORDS. AIDS, crystal, gay, HIV, HIV prevention, homosexuality, Internet research, men who have sex with men (MSM), methamphetamine, STI, substance use, unprotected anal intercourse (UAI)

INTRODUCTION

Crystal methamphetamine (crystal) use among men who have sex with men (MSM) has been on the rise, and its relationship to high-risk sexual behavior, and consequently HIV risk, has received recent research (Halkitis et al., 2001; Reback and Ditman, 1997; Semple et al., 2002) and media attention (Halkitis & Galatowitsch, 2004; Owen, 2004; Reuters, 2004). With an 11% increase in the number of newly diagnosed HIV infections among MSM between 2000 and 2003 (CDC, 2004), a better understanding of crystal and other drug use in connection with high-risk behavior is needed. Previous research has indicated that crystal use is associated with "marathon sex" (prolonged sexual activity) and unprotected anal intercourse (UAI) (Reback and Ditman, 1997; Semple et al., 2002; Whittington et al., 2002).

Medical and Health Research Association of New York City, Inc. (MHRA), in collaboration with the New York State Psychiatric Institute, Columbia University (NYSPI/CU) and the Centers for Disease Control and Prevention (CDC), conducted two national Internet-based surveys of high-risk sexual behavior among MSM. Data from these surveys were analyzed to better understand the relationship between substance use and UAI. As the majority of research on HIV and risk behavior has been conducted in small geographic areas or within cities where HIV is endemic (Leigh and Stall, 1993), this overview will describe differing levels of crystal use across U.S. regions and associations found between substance use and unprotected sex among MSM recruited online.

METHODS

Both Internet studies were anonymous and cross-sectional, inquiring about sexual and drug-using behaviors among MSM. The surveys were linked to online recruitment banners that were posted on participating websites. Both surveys included information on demographics (age group, race/ethnicity, education, income and residence), and assessment of risk behaviors, such as type of sexual contact (anal, oral, vaginal–each with and without condoms), knowledge of respondents' HIV status, knowledge of partners' HIV status, type of illicit drug use, frequency of alcohol consumption, whether drugs or alcohol were used before or during sex, and how sex partners were met. No personally identifying information was collected. For *Study 1,* year of birth and the first three digits of the zip code were obtained. For *Study 2,* year of birth and the state and country of residence were obtained. Links to STI/HIV prevention and treatment websites and mental health hotlines appeared at the end of each survey. Survey questions were adapted from questionnaires used by the investigators in previous studies.

Study participation for both studies was limited to men 18 and older, and all participants clicked on an online consent form before gaining access to the survey. The surveys neither used cookies nor collected user IP addresses with submitted data. Both surveys received Institutional Review Board approval (*Study 1:* MHRA and NYSPI/CU. *Study 2:* MHRA, CDC and NYSPI/CU). There were no monetary incentives to complete either survey.

Study 1

Participants were recruited from one general interest, gay-oriented site between June and July 2002. The survey inquired about behaviors during a recent 6-month period. Analysis was limited to 2,915 men who reported sex with other men or who self-identified as gay or bisexual. Survey questions addressed drug and sex behaviors occurring within this 6-month period and did not focus on any particular sexual encounter. Detailed reports on drug use and sexually transmitted diseases from this study have been reported elsewhere (Hirshfield Remien, Humberstone et al., 2004; Hirshfield, Remien, Walavalkar et al., 2004).

Study 2

Participants were recruited between October and March 2003-2004 from 14 gay-oriented sites, ranging from general news, to chat, to commercial sex sites. This study built on the research and technological experience of *Study 1* and was multidimensional. The respondent's answers to questions dictated the course of the survey. For example, if the respondent met his last sex partner online, he would see questions about meeting people online, whereas if the respondent met his last partner offline, he would not see these particular questions. The goal of this study was to elicit information on the last sexual encounter within the past 3 months. The survey collected data on participants' last sexual encounter, as well as the demographic and behavioral information mentioned above. Analysis was limited to the 2,770 men from the United States or Canada who self-identified as gay or bisexual or reported oral or anal sex with a man within three months prior to the survey.

RESULTS

Participants in *Studies 1* and *2* were similar with regard to race/ethnicity, sexual orientation, HIV prevalence and regional use of crystal. Both samples were predominately white (80%). Most men reported having sex only with men. The self-reported HIV prevalence of both samples was 7%. Both studies found a strong association between crystal use and UAI despite differing study time frames (*Study 1*, 81% of crystal users reported UAI vs. 55% of non-users; *Study 2*, 81% of crystal users reported UAI vs. 54% of non-users).

Crystal use was reported significantly more in the western U.S. than eastern in both studies. In *Study 1*, 6% of the overall sample reported crystal use during the six-month study period. The Pacific and Mountain regions each had a 7% higher reporting of crystal use than the Northeast region and a 6% higher reporting than the North Central region (Pacific regional difference, $p \leq .01$; Mountain regional difference, $p \leq .05$). In *Study 2*, 3% of the overall sample reported crystal use in their last sexual encounter. Crystal use was reported more in the Pacific region than any other U.S. region (a range of 6%-8% higher; $p \leq .001$ for all regions).

Study 1

Participants resided in all fifty states, roughly in proportion to the population of each state. Nearly half were between 18 and 30 years of age, with a range of 18 to 83. Most reported up to $40,000 income and some college education or more. About 80% reported meeting sex partners online. The number of lifetime sex partners ranged from 0 to over 1,000, with about one quarter of the participants reporting more than 100 life-time partners. The majority reported more than one sex partner during the six-month study period. About one-third of the overall sample reported any drug or alcohol use before or during sex.

Demographic differences were found between crystal and non-crystal users. Men aged 40 and over were significantly less likely to report crystal use than men aged 18-24 (p < .01), men aged 25-29 (p < .01), or men aged 30-39 (p < .05). Crystal use was also reported significantly less among men with some college education or more (p < .01) and those earning over $40,000 (p = .001). There were no differences by race/ethnicity.

Compared to those not reporting crystal during the study period, crystal users were significantly more likely to report polydrug use (two or more drugs), alcohol before or during sex, UAI, and any sexually transmitted infection (STI). Of note, 82% of crystal users reported having UAI at least once in the six months before taking the survey, compared to 55% of the non-crystal users. Additionally, 93% of crystal users reported a range of 2-100+ partners in the prior six months compared to 79% of non-crystal users. The most common drugs also reported by crystal users were marijuana, ecstasy, poppers, cocaine, and Viagra. Crystal users were somewhat more likely to be HIV-positive than non-users (p = .07).

Study 2

Participants were from all 50 U.S. states and Canada. Nearly half were between ages 18 and 35, with a range of 18 to 85. Slightly more than half earned over $40,000 per year. Half had a college degree or more. The number of lifetime sex partners ranged from 1 to over 1,000, with 30% of participants reporting over 100 lifetime partners. In the three months prior to the survey, respondents reported a range of 0 to 150 male partners. Fifty-four percent reported anal sex in their last encounter; of those, 56% reported UAI. Roughly equal proportions met their last partner online (51%) and offline (49%). About 20% reported drug or alcohol use before or during their last sexual encounter.

In the three months prior to the survey, crystal users reported a range of 0 to 130 sex partners, with a median of 6, while non-crystal users reported a range of 0 to 150 partners with a median of 2. There was no difference in use by race/ethnicity, income, or education. However, men aged 30-39 years were significantly more likely to report crystal (p < .05) than men aged 18-24 and men 40 years or older.

Main comparisons between crystal and non-crystal users found that, in the last encounter, crystal users were significantly more likely to report engaging in receptive UAI, binge drinking (5 or more drinks) or using Viagra before or during sex, polydrug use, and being diagnosed with an STI since this last sexual encounter. Additionally, crystal users were significantly more likely to be a commercial sex worker and to be HIV positive than non-users (p < .001). Most crystal users reported anal sex in their last encounter (82%); of those, 83% exchanged money or drugs for UAI. The most common drugs used in the same encounter with crystal were Viagra, poppers, Gamma Hydroxy Butyrate (GHB), ecstasy, and marijuana. Although crystal users and non-users were similar in their "yes/no" responses about wanting to learn more about HIV or prevention online, crystal users were significantly more likely than non-users to report that they were "not sure" if they wanted to learn more about these topics (22% versus 13%, p < .01).

DISCUSSION

Conducting *Studies 1 and 2* via the Internet enabled us to recruit participants from all U.S. states, including smaller cities and rural areas, which are missed in behavioral surveys that typically recruit from large cities. The high-risk drug use and sexual behaviors found in *Studies 1 and 2* confirm previous research (using traditional methods) on crystal use among MSM, which indicates that it is associated with young age, having a greater number of sex partners, having unprotected anal intercourse, having an STI, and being HIV-positive (Molitor et al., 1998; Reback and Ditman, 1997; Semple et al., 2002, 2003). Further, the rate of unprotected anal intercourse among crystal users was nearly identical across *Studies 1 and 2*. This consistency may indicate a common pattern of drug use and sexual behavior. The similarity of findings from our Internet-based surveys to those using more traditional forms of recruitment and interview methods suggests that online surveys are a reliable way to study high-risk sexual behavior in MSM.

Although the proportion of MSM who reported crystal use in *Studies 1 and 2* was relatively small, crystal users were significantly more likely than non-users to report unprotected sex, potentially putting them at risk for HIV and other STIs (Halkitis et al., 2001; Reback and Ditman, 1997; Semple et al., 2002).

Crystal use among MSM has been an increasing public health concern in the western U.S. since the early 1990s (Halkitis et al., 2001; Semple et al., 2003). Regional findings from *Studies 1 and 2* indicate that the highest reporting of crystal use was found in the Pacific region, where it has historically been most prevalent (Sullivan et al., 1998; Thiede et al., 2003). According to a recent national report (NIDA, 2003), indicators of methamphetamine use remained highest in Pacific and Mountain regions. Relatively low indicators of crystal abuse were found in North East and South Atlantic regions. However, reports of crystal use in MSM in the North East appear to be on the rise (Halkitis, 2004; Owen, 2004; Reuters, 2004).

Some limitations of these studies deserve mention. Since both surveys were anonymous, we could neither verify the reliability of respondents' identities nor their responses. In *Study 1*, we could not link risk behavior to any specific encounter. In *Study 2*, we had only one event to base sexual and drug information upon and therefore could not detect a pattern of behavior. In both studies, we did not collect information on the level and frequency of current or past drug use (and context of use). Further, we cannot determine from these Internet studies whether the men that participated are representative of the population of MSM using the Internet, of MSM in general, or of MSM with HIV, since the MSM population has never been enumerated. Nevertheless, Internet research is an efficient and inexpensive way to reach large samples of high-risk groups.

Studies conducted over the past 20 years have found associations between substance abuse treatment and a reduction in HIV risk behaviors (Metzger and Navaline, 2003). There are challenges to treating crystal abuse; drug treatment must focus on helping men addicted to crystal re-learn to have sex without it (Frosch et al., 1996). There is a need for greater integration of substance use education and treatment into HIV prevention and care. Ongoing drug surveillance is necessary to document new trends in substance use patterns among MSM (Stall et al., 2001) in order to create multifaceted interventions. This study's ability to quickly reach large numbers of men reporting high-risk behaviors demonstrates the potential for online HIV education, prevention, and outreach.

REFERENCES

Centers for Disease Control (2004), Diagnoses of HIV/AIDS–32 states, 2000-2003. *Morbidity & Mortality Weekly Report*, 53:1106-1110.

Frosch, D., Shoptaw, S., Huber, A., Rawson, R. & Ling, W. (1996), Sexual HIV risk among gay and bisexual male methamphetamine abusers. *J. Substance Abuse Treatment*, 13:483-486.

Halkitis, P. (2004), *The Crystal Meth-HIV Connection*. Paper presented at the HIV Forum NYC, New York, February 28.

Halkitis, P. & Galatowitsch, P. (2004), Crystal-meth is about to race out of control. *Newsday*, p. A39, March 9.

Halkitis, P., Parsons, J. & Stirratt, M. (2001) A double epidemic: Crystal methamphetamine drug use in relation to HIV transmission among gay men. *J. Homosexuality*, 41:17-35.

Hirshfield, S., Remien, R., Humberstone, M., Walavalkar, I. & Chiasson, M. (2004), Substance use and high-risk sex among men who have sex with men: A national on-line study in the USA. *AIDS Care*, 16:1036-1047.

Hirshfield, S., Remien, R., Walavalkar, I. & Ma, C. (2004). Crystal methamphetamine use predicts incident STD infection among men who have sex with men: A nested case-control study. *J. Medical Internet Research*, 6:e41.

Leigh, B. & Stall, R. (1993), Substance use and risky sexual behavior for exposure to HIV. Issues in methodology, interpretation, and prevention. *American Psychologist*, 48:1035-1045.

Metzger, D. & Navaline, H. (2003), Human Immunodeficiency Virus prevention and the potential of drug abuse treatment. *Clinical Infectious Diseases*, 37:s451-s456.

Molitor, F., Truax, S., Ruiz, J. & Sun, R. (1998), Association of methamphetamine use during sex with risky sexual behaviors and HIV infection among non-injection drug users. *Western J. Medicine*, 168:93-97.

NIDA (2003), *Epidemiologic Trends in Drug Abuse*. National Institute of Drug Abuse, Community Epidemiology Work Group.

Owen, F. (2004). No man is a crystal meth user unto himself. *New York Times*, pp. 1,10, August 29.

Reback, C. & Ditman, D. (1997), *The Social Construction of a Gay Drug: Methamphetamine Use Among Gay and Bisexual Males in Los Angeles. Executive Summary*. City of Los Angeles, AIDS Coordinator. Los Angeles.

Reuters (2004), Crystal meth linked to AIDS in New York: "Party" drug increases HIV risk among gays. *MSNBC*, http://www.msnbc.msn.com/id/5158153/.

Semple, S., Patterson, T. & Grant, I. (2002), Motivations associated with methamphetamine use among HIV+ men who have sex with men. *J. Substance Abuse Treatment*, 22:149-156.

Semple, S., Patterson, T. & Grant, I. (2003), Binge use of methamphetamine among HIV-positive men who have sex with men: Pilot data and HIV prevention implications. *AIDS Education & Prevention*, 15:133-147.

Stall, R., Paul, J., Greenwood, G., Pollack, L., Bein, E., Crosby, G., Mills, T., Binson, D., Coates, T. & Catania, J. (2001), Alcohol use, drug use and alcohol-related problems among men who have sex with men: The Urban Men's Health Study. *Addiction*, 96:1589-1601.

Sullivan, P., Nakashima, A., Purcell, D. & Waard, J. (1998), Geographic differences in noninjection and injection substance use among HIV-seropositive men who have sex with men: western United States versus other regions. Supplement to HIV/AIDS Surveillance Study Group. *J. Acquired Immune Deficiency Syndrome*, 19:266-273.

Thiede, H., Valleroy, L., Mackellar, D., Celentano, D., Ford, W., Hagan, H., Koblin, B., LaLota, M., McFarland, W., Shehan, D. & Torian, L. (2003), Regional patterns and correlates of substance use among young men who have sex with men in 7 US urban areas. *American J. Public Health*, 93:1915-1921.

Whittington, W., Collis, T., Dithmer-Schreck, D., Handsfield, H., Shalit, P., Wood, R., Holmes, K. & Celum, C. (2002), Sexually transmitted diseases and human immunodeficiency virus–Discordant partnerships among men who have sex with men. *Clinical Infectious Diseases*, 35:1010-1017.

Methamphetamine Use, Sexual Behavior, and HIV Seroconversion

Perry N. Halkitis, PhD
Kelly A. Green, MPH
Daniel J. Carragher, PhD

SUMMARY. Methamphetamine use has been closely linked to sexual risk taking in the gay and bisexual population. While previous studies have noted this relationship, few empirical investigations have quantified this association. As part of a larger, longitudinal study of club drug use among gay and bisexual men in New York City, the authors assessed the sexual risk taking of those who identified as methamphetamine users. A subset of these men, who reported either a seronegative or unknown HIV status, was confirmed to be HIV-positive. Comparisons of this group to confirmed HIV-negative methamphetamine using men in this study's sample indicated that these not known to be HIV positive individuals differed in their reasons for methamphetamine use and in terms of their sexual risk taking. In particular, those who had seroconverted reported higher levels of unprotected receptive anal in-

Perry N. Halkitis is Professor and Director of the Center for Health, Identity, Behavior & Prevention Studies (CHIBPS), Department of Applied Psychology, New York University.

Kelly A. Green was a graduate student of Applied Psychology and Research Associate, and Daniel J. Carragher is Senior Research Scientist, CHIBPS.

Address correspondence to: Perry N. Halkitis, 82 Washington Square East, Suite 553, New York, NY 10003.

[Haworth co-indexing entry note]: "Methamphetamine Use, Sexual Behavior, and HIV Seroconversion." Halkitis, Perry N., Kelly A. Green, and Daniel J. Carragher. Co-published simultaneously in *Journal of Gay & Lesbian Psychotherapy* (The Haworth Medical Press, an imprint of The Haworth Press, Inc.) Vol. 10, No. 3/4, 2006, pp. 95-109; and: *Crystal Meth and Men Who Have Sex with Men: What Mental Health Care Professionals Need to Know* (ed: Milton L. Wainberg, Andrew J. Kolodny, and Jack Drescher) The Haworth Medical Press, an imprint of The Haworth Press, Inc., 2006, pp. 95-109. Single or multiple copies of this article are available for a fee from The Haworth Document Delivery Service [1-800-HAWORTH, 9:00 a.m. - 5:00 p.m. (EST). E-mail address: docdelivery@haworthpress.com].

tercourse while high. Our study confirms that methamphetamine may play a causal role in HIV infection and may fuel the HIV epidemic at large. *[Article copies available for a fee from The Haworth Document Delivery Service: 1-800-HAWORTH. E-mail address: <docdelivery@haworthpress.com> Website: <http://www.HaworthPress.com> © 2006 by The Haworth Press, Inc. All rights reserved.]*

KEYWORDS. Gay, HIV, homosexual, men who have sex with men (MSM), methamphetamine, seroconversion, sexually transmitted infections (STIs), sexual risk taking

The use and abuse of methamphetamine by men-who-have-sex-with-men (MSM) in New York City (NYC) has risen sharply in the last several years and has created the potential for a methamphetamine epidemic. Previously, the problem has been minimal when compared to the abuse of the substance in the Midwestern and Western parts of the United States (Halkitis, Parsons and Stirratt, 2001; Rawson, Gonzales and Brethen, 2002). However, recently, methamphetamine has become a common element in dance clubs, bars, commercial sex environments, and circuit parties/raves in NYC, and is often taken in conjunction with other recreational drugs and/or alcohol (Halkitis, Green and Mourgues, 2005; Halkitis, Parsons and Wilton, 2003).

The health risks associated with methamphetamine use stem from two sources: the methamphetamine addiction itself and the potential transmission of Human Immunodeficiency Virus (HIV) or other sexually transmitted infections (STIs) which are facilitated due to the intimate link that exists between methamphetamine use and sexual risk taking. In effect, a "double epidemic" is possible (Halkitis, Parsons and Stirratt, 2001; Halkitis, Fischgrund and Parsons, 2005; Halkitis, Shrem and Martin, 2005; Reback, 1997).

The potential for increased methamphetamine use among MSM in NYC presents dangerous implications for efforts to fight the HIV/AIDS epidemic (Halkitis, Parsons and Stirratt, 2001; Harris et al., 1993; Reback, 1997; Sorvillo et al., 1995). Methamphetamine use is highly associated with sexual risk taking in MSM (Guss, 2000; Semple et al., 2002) and in NYC, where 25% of those living with HIV or AIDS are MSM (New York City Department of Health, 2002), methamphetamine use could seriously compromise primary and secondary efforts to prevent HIV transmission as well as exacerbate the transmission of other

STIs such as syphilis and gonorrhea, which have recently escalated in NYC among MSM (Centers for Disease Control and Prevention, 2000; de Luise et al., 2000). Secondly, use of methamphetamine can create serious health consequences for HIV-positive individuals by not only undermining health related behaviors such as HIV medication adherence, but also by affecting the health of organ systems that are already ravaged by HIV.

Research has shown that the association between methamphetamine use and sexual risk taking is most pronounced among MSM (Frosch et al., 1996; Halkitis and Parsons, 2002; Reback, 1997; Semple et al., 2002), including ethnic and racial minorities (Nemoto, Operario and Soma, 2002). This relationship is exacerbated by the context in which the drug is used by many MSM, such as commercial sex environments (Parsons and Halkitis, 2002), where the use of the substance occurs within the context of a highly sexualized arena. As methamphetamine creates a sense of euphoria, many MSM use the drug as a means of heightening their sexual behavior (Ellenhorn et al., 1997; Halkitis, Parsons and Stirratt, 2001).

Methamphetamine use, when coupled with high-risk sexual behavior, foretells that the growing use of the drug in NYC is certain to exacerbate the HIV/AIDS epidemic. Further, the synergy between the methamphetamine and HIV epidemics is heightened when methamphetamine is injected (Bull, Rietmeijer and Piper, 2002).

Thus, the purpose of this study's analysis is to describe the methamphetamine and sexual risk behaviors of a cohort of gay and bisexual men in New York City. Specifically, we sought to characterize this drug-sex link in a subset of men who self-reported being HIV-negative but who were detected to be HIV seropositive.

METHODS

Design

Project BUMPS (Boys Using Multiple Party Substances) was a year-long longitudinal study of 450 gay and bisexual club drug-using men. The aims of the study were to evaluate developmental trajectories in club drug use and sexual risk taking, as well as the relationships between these trajectories. For the purposes of this study, club drugs were defined as one of the five following illicit substances: gamma-hydroxybutyrate (GHB), ketamine, 3,4-Methylene Dioxy Methamphetamine (MDMA; "Ecstasy"), methamphetamine, and powdered cocaine.

Participants were recruited between February 2001 and October 2002 in NYC using active and passive techniques in venues frequented by gay and bisexual men, such as bars, bathhouses, dance clubs, and community sites.

Eligibility criteria for this study included: (1) being 18 years of age or older; (2) self-identifying as gay or bisexual; (3) being biologically male; and (4) indicating six instances of club drug use in the year prior to screening, with at least one instance of use in combination with male-to-male sex in the previous six months.

Those who met the eligibility criteria were scheduled for a baseline interview where study consent was obtained and both qualitative and quantitative data collection took place. Men were followed at three more assessment points–4, 8, and 12 months post-baseline.

At the baseline assessment HIV status was confirmed. Those who self-reported a seropositive status provided proof of this status (i.e., doctor's letter, prescription bottle with participant's name, etc.). Those who self-reported as seronegative or unknown HIV status underwent mandatory HIV antibody testing via the OraSure system to test for oral HIV antibodies. At the final assessment (12 months post baseline) voluntary testing was encouraged for all those who tested seronegative at baseline.

Participants received an incentive for each assessment that they completed. All procedures were approved by the IRB of New York University.

Measures

Reported here is a subset of the quantitative measures utilized at the baseline assessment, which was administered via the Audio Computer-Assisted Self Interview (ACASI).

Sociodemographics. Participants were asked to self-report their age, race/ethnicity, HIV serostatus, education level, employment status, income, and sexual orientation identification. In addition, as noted earlier HIV status was confirmed.

Club Drug Use. Club drug use was measured via a version of a scale developed for a previous study by the investigative team (Halkitis, Parsons and Wilton, 2003). This scale assesses the frequency (as defined by days of use) of each of the five club drugs used over a period of 4 months prior to the interview, as well as the incidence of usage in relation to sexual activity during the same 4-month period. On this scale, individuals are asked to provide frequency of use in two ways: on a five-point Likert scale (ranging from "never" to "always") and on a ratio scale, recording the number of days the drugs had been used. In addition, participants were asked to identify other illicit drugs that had been used in conjunction with each of the club drugs via a checklist for the period of assessment.

Reasons for Methamphetamine Use. To assess reasons for use, we utilized the *Inventory of Methamphetamine Using Situations.* This measure consisted of 35 items modified from *The Inventory of Drug Taking Situations* (IDTS) (Annis, Turner and Sklar, 1996). Participants were asked to respond using a 5-point Likert scale, ranging from "Never" to "Always," indicating how often they had used methamphetamine under various situations during the past three months. The measure included five subscales (Unpleasant Emotions, Physical Discomfort, Conflict with Others, Social Pressure, and Pleasant Times with Others) reflecting categories of situations under which drug use might occur (alphas ranged from .73 to .95).

Sexual Behavior. We used three pre-established scales to measure sexual activity with primary partners, and with non-primary or "casual" partners who are HIV-positive, HIV-negative, or HIV-status unknown. These scales, *Sexual Relationships and Activities Scale* (SRAS), *Sexual Activity Primary Partner Scale* (SAPPS), and *Sexual Activity Other Partners Scale* (SAOPS), assessed the number of different male sexual partners in the 4-month period of assessment, as well as the frequency of sexual activities and of sexual behaviors with each of the two partner types (primary and non-primary) as well as across varying serostatus (HIV-positive, HIV-negative, and status unknown) non-primary partners. In addition, we assessed each of these behaviors while under the influence of any of the club drugs.

RESULTS

At baseline, 450 men were recruited and assessed. On average, these men were 33-years-old (SD = 7.93), and ranged in age from 18 to 67. About half the sample were men of color. Similar levels of diversity were noted in terms of their self-reported HIV status, educational attainment, work status, and annual income. In terms of sexual orientation, 88% (n = 396) identified as gay and the remainder (n = 54) as bisexual. Of these 54 bisexual men, more than half (n = 29) indicated sex with a woman in period of assessment. A further description of the sample is shown in Table 1.

TABLE 1. Participant Characteristics in Project BUMPS (N = 450)

	n	%
Race/Ethnicity		
African American	66	14.7
Latino/Hispanic	89	19.8
White	230	51.1
Other	65	14.4
Sexual Orientation		
Gay/Homosexual	396	88.0
Bisexual	54	12.0
Educational Background		
H.S. Degree or less	64	14.2
Some College/Associates	155	34.4
Bachelors Degree	165	36.7
Graduate Degree	66	14.7
Employment Status		
Employed Full Time	170	37.8
Employed Part Time	104	23.1
Permanently Disabled	51	11.3
Unemployed	124	27.6
Missing	1	0.2
Annual Income		
Less than $10,000/yr	77	17.1
$10,000-$39,999/yr	209	46.4
$40,000-$74,999/yr	119	26.4
More than $75,000/yr	39	8.7
Missing	6	1.3

All 150 men who self-reported being HIV-positive at baseline were confirmed as such. Of the 274 self-reported HIV-negative men, 11 (4%) actually tested HIV-positive at baseline; also, of the 26 men who indicated that they were unaware of their HIV status, 5 (19.2%) tested HIV-positive. These 16 unknown to be HIV positive men were diverse in terms of their race/ethnicity. Among the 11 men who reported an HIV-negative status and tested seropositive, 4 (36.4%) were African American, 4 (36.4%) were White, 2 (18.2%) were Latino, and 1 (9.1%) was of mixed race. Similarly, among the 5 self-reported unknown status men, 3 (60%) of the seroconverts were African American while 2 (40%) were White.

Comparisons of the 16 seroconverts to those who were confirmed to be HIV-negative, indicate that these men were not significantly or practically different in terms of age (29 years-old vs. 31-years-old) or annual income than those who tested negative at baseline. However, testing seropositive at baseline was related to race ($\chi^2(3) = 18.66$, $p < .001$), and marginally related to educational attainment ($\chi^2(3) = 8.19$, $p = .04$), although the relationship between race and education attainment confounds this finding ($\chi^2(9) = 40.92$, $p < .001$). Specifically, of the 33 African-American men tested for HIV antibodies at baseline, 21.2% tested positive, as compared to only 3.7% of the White men, 3.4% of the Latino men, and 2.2% of men grouped as Other race/ethnicity. These data are further shown in Table 2.

TABLE 2. Comparison of Confirmed HIV-Negative vs. Seroconverts at Baseline

	Seroconverts		HIV-Negative	
	n	%	n	%
Race/Ethnicity*				
African American	7	43.8	26	9.2
Latino/Hispanic	2	37.5	56	19.7
White	6	12.5	157	55.3
Other	1	6.2	45	15.8
Educational Background**				
H.S. Degree or less	2	12.5	35	12.3
Some College/Associates	10	62.5	84	29.6
Bachelors Degree	3	18.8	121	42.6
Graduate Degree	1	6.2	44	15.5

*p < 0.001
**p < 0.05

Methamphetamine Use Among Seroconverts

Of the 450 men in this sample, 65% (n = 293) indicated that they had used methamphetamine in the four months prior to assessment. Further information on the methamphetamine using behaviors of the BUMPS sample can be seen in Halkitis, Green and Mourgues (2005). In terms of methamphetamine use, the 16 seroconverts were as likely as those who tested HIV-negative at baseline to have reported use of the substance (63% vs. 64%, respectively). Specifically, of these 293 methamphetamine using-men, 192 indicated that they were HIV-negative or status unknown at baseline, and of these 10 tested HIV-positive (here forth referred to as seroconverts) while the remaining 182 were confirmed to actually be HIV-negative. Among this subset of methamphetamine users, the number of days that the seroconverts used the substance in the four months prior to assessment was equivalent statistically to those who tested HIV-negative at baseline, although qualitatively the seroconverts reported 18 days of use in the previous four months while the others reported only 12 days of use.

Since poly-drug use is a common phenomenon among club drug using gay and bisexual men (Halkitis, Green and Mourgues, 2005), we next assessed the other substance that the men used in combination with methamphetamine. The seroconverts and the confirmed HIV-negative men were just as likely to combine their methamphetamine with cocaine, ketamine, GHB, MDMA, alcohol, marijuana, inhalant nitrates, and Viagra. Among the 10 seroconverts, the percentage of men indicating combination of methamphetamine with other substances was as follows: alcohol (70%, n = 7), MDMA (50%, n = 5), GHB (40%, n = 4), ketamine (40%, n = 4), marijuana (40%, n = 4), inhalant nitrates (30%, n = 3), cocaine (28.6%, n = 2), and Viagra (10%, n = 1).

Finally, an assessment was made of the reasons why the methamphetamine users indicated that they partook of the substance; this was based on the scale developed by Anis, Turner and Sklar (1996). These data are shown in Table 3 and indicate the seroconverts endorse most of the reasons for use at higher levels than those who were confirmed to be HIV-negative, yet only significantly greater when indicating their reasons for use were to avoid physical discomfort (t(190) = 3.00, $p < .01$), and tangentially to avoid conflict (t(190) = 1.86, $p = .09$) and to have pleasant times with others (t(190) = 1.66, $p = .10$).

TABLE 3. Reasons for Methamphetamine Use

	Seroconverts		HIV-Negative	
	Mean	SD	Mean	SD
Avoid unpleasant emotions	22.70	14.11	18.03	10.11
Avoid physical discomfort*	11.90	3.78	8.54	3.43
Avoid conflict with others**	20.00	10.49	13.73	7.31
Social pressures	9.50	2.99	9.81	4.67
Pleasant times with others***	17.00	6.58	14.30	4.91

*p < 0.01
**p = 0.09
***p = 0.10

Sexual Behavior of Methamphetamine Using Seroconverts

In the overall sample of 450, men who reported the use of methamphetamine also indicated a greater number of male sexual partners in the 4-month period of assessment than those who indicated no use of the substance (t(447) = 4.89, p < .001). The methamphetamine users reported an average of 20 (SD = 28.34) partners in the period of assessment, while the non-users reported only 10 (SD = 15.42) partners.

Furthermore, all of the 10 seroconverts and 182 confirmed HIV-negative methamphetamine-using men indicated they had engaged in sexual behavior in the 4 months prior to assessment. Moreover, this sample reported an average of 17 (SD = 23.85) different male sexual partners, with a median value of 9, and arrange of 1-200. Interestingly, the seroconverts reported the same number of sexual partners as the non-seroconverts in the period of assessment.

Primary Partner Sexual Behavior. With regard to primary sexual partners (i.e., boyfriends, lovers, etc.), 54.9% (n = 100) of those who were confirmed to be negative at baseline also indicated being in a relationship, while only 20% (n = 2) of the seroconverts reported this status, although this does not reach significance based on the continuity correction of the chi-square analysis. Interestingly, while the majority of the 182 of the confirmed HIV negative men (87.6%) reported a seroconcordant partner, both of the partnered seroconverts indicated that they had not discussed serostatus with their primary partners. Analysis of specific sexual acts were nor undertaken given the limited sample size of those seroconverts in primary partner relationships.

Non-Primary Partner Sexual Behavior. Among the methamphetamine using sub-sample, the seroconverts were just as likely as those confirmed to be HIV-negative to report sex with a non-primary partner in the period of assessment. Specifically, 87.4% (n = 159) of the confirmed negative men reported sex with these types of partners while 90% of the seroconverts reported sex with non-primary partners. Furthermore, the seroconverts and confirmed HIV-negative men reported an equivalent number of non-primary partners (17 and 16, respectively). Although statistical significance was not achieved, the seroconverts also reported more occasions in which they had engaged in group sex than those confirmed to be HIV-negative (7 vs. 4 occasions, respectively).

Finally, we assessed the frequency to which these 192 methamphetamine-using men engaged in unprotected receptive anal intercourse (URAI), the riskiest of HIV transmission behaviors (Vittinghoff et al., 1999), with non-primary partners. We sought to disentangle whether the frequency of this behavior varied in situations in which the participants were high vs. not high and across the two groups of men (i.e., seroconverts vs. confirmed HIV-negative). Our multivariate model reached significance indicating that the men reported more occasions of URAI while high as compared to not high ($F(1, 183) = 919.80, p < .001$). Specifically, men reported an average of 2.47 (SD = 10.64) acts while high as compared to 1.67 (SD = 7.70) acts while not high. Furthermore, the seroconverts reported much higher rates of URAI than the confirmed HIV-negative men while high ($F(1, 183) = 894/31, p < 001$). Specifically, while the seroconverts reported an average of 18.78 (SD = 33.00) while high, the confirmed HIV-negative men reported 1.64 (SD = 7.43) such acts when high. Rates of URAI were equivalent across the two groups while not high. These data are further illustrated in Figure 1.

DISCUSSION

As has been noted in the literature for some time, the connection between methamphetamine use and sexual risk taking is a pernicious one. The substance may act as a facilitator, which psychologically disinhibits its users, undermines safer sex strategies, and exacerbates HIV infection. It may be that methamphetamine is a particular type of drug, because of the hypersexual and euphoric states it induces, that also provides a type of cognitive escape (McKirnan, Ostrow and Hope, 1996) resulting in greater risk taking. Whether this relationship between use of the drug and sexual risk behavior among gay and bisexual men is a direct one is un-

FIGURE 1. Frequency of URAI

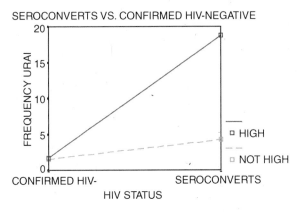

SEROCONVERTS VS. CONFIRMED HIV-NEGATIVE

URAI: Unprotected receptive anal intercourse

clear. What is more likely is that men with certain psychological profiles are attracted to methamphetamine, use it in environments and contexts that are sexually charged (Parsons and Halkitis, 2002), and as a result are situated to engage in sexual risk. Whether men use the drug intentionally as a way to facilitate sexual risk taking behavior or whether sexual risk taking is a natural byproduct of methamphetamine use are issues that need to be further disentangled. Regardless of the actual manifestations of these relationships, the fact remains that among methamphetamine using gay and bisexual men, studies have shown that many of these men are HIV-positive (Reback, 1997; Shoptaw, Reback and Freese, 2002) and thus use of the drug among the seropositive is likely to be associated with sexual risk taking which may lead to new HIV infections in this population.

What is clear, however, from the results of this study, is that methamphetamine use, as has been previously shown (Halkitis, Parsons and Wilton, 2003; Mansergh et al., 2001; Mattison et al., 2001; Woody et al., 2001), is endemic to urban gay and bisexual men, which concurrently are HIV epicenters. Our data clearly indicate that use of methamphetamine is associated with higher levels of sexual risk taking, more specifically showing that unprotected receptive anal intercourse is more likely to occur when an individual is high than when he is not high. Furthermore, in comparisons of men unknown to be HIV positive in this study (seroconverts) to those who were confirmed to be HIV-negative, rates of unprotected receptive anal intercourse were markedly higher when methamphetamine was being used. Consistent with previous work (Greenwood et al., 2000), methamphetamine users reported significantly more sexual partners than non-users, thus increasing the probability of infection simply because of the greater number of men with whom they engage in sex. Finally, our findings also support the idea that the use of methamphetamine may facilitate higher risk sexual activities that may not occur when one is not using the drug. This is further supported by the fact that those in this study who were not aware of their HIV positive status reported higher levels of use of the drug for social pleasure.

Not surprisingly, this study also indicates that among those who had seroconverted, use of methamphetamine with other substances was not uncommon. Poly-drug use has been noted previously in the methamphetamine-using population (Halkitis, Parsons and Wilton, 2003), although interestingly, only one of this study's seroconverts reported using methamphetamine with Viagra. As has been noted (Halkitis, Parsons and Stirratt, 2001), methamphetamine use causes erectile dysfunction, and thus the relatively low use of Viagra among the seroconverts in this study suggests that perhaps they are more likely to engage in the anal receptive role while high on methamphetamine, thus increasing the likelihood of HIV infection.

As will all self-report based studies, these findings should be viewed with caution. However, the administration of the surveys via ACASI, as well as the trust that our research team possesses with the gay male community of New York City, function to counterbalance the problems associated with self-reports of high risk behaviors. Further, the relatively small sub-sample of men who had seroconverted presented a challenge in our statistical analysis. Nonetheless, the fact that some relationships are established, are done so powerfully, and are in line with previous findings regarding methamphetamine use in the gay and bisexual male community, suggests a certain level of trust in the knowledge that is generated here. Even though precise timing of primary HIV infection was not established in the 16 unknown to be HIV positive individuals who seroconverted in our study, having a better understanding of them may help develop more effective prevention strategies as they may represent those who "efficiently" expose themselves to more sexual risk behaviors and get infected with HIV.

In the end, the work presented here speaks to the attention that needs to be given to the ever-growing methamphetamine problem in the gay and bisexual male communities of the United States. Clinicians working with this population need to consider the level of use of the drug among their clients, and initiate interventions that seek to capture and address the reasons and context of use of methamphetamine. A holistic understanding of the use of this drug nested within the lives of these men will more likely lead to intervention strategies that consider the role of the drug in relation to sex, as well as the psychological states of gay and bisexual men. Ultimately, we must seek to avert the continued use of methamphetamine in the gay and bisexual community, as ongoing use is likely to exacerbate both the HIV and drug abuse epidemic.

REFERENCES

Annis, H.M., Turner, N.E. & Sklar, S.M. (1996), *Inventory of Drug-Taking Situations: User's Guide*. Toronto, Ontario: Addiction Research Foundation.

Bull, S., Rietmeijer C. & Piper P. (2001), Synergistic risk for HIV: The complexity of behavior among men who have sex with men and also inject drugs. *J. Homosexuality*, 42:29-49.

Centers for Disease Control and Prevention (CDC) (2000), *Consultation on Recent Trends in STD and HIV Morbidity and Risk Behaviors Among MSM. Meeting Report*. Atlanta, GA: Author, October 30-31.

de Luise, C., Brown, J., Rubin, S. & Blank, S. (2000), *Emerging Patterns in Primary and Secondary Syphilis Among Men: NYC: January-September 2000*. New York City: Author.

Ellenhorn, M.J., Schonwald, S., Ordog, G. & Wasserberger, J. (1997), *Ellenhorn's Medical Toxicology: Diagnosis and Treatment of Human Poisoning*. (2nd ed.). Baltimore: Williams & Wilkins.

Frosch, D., Shoptaw, S., Huber, A., Rawson, R.A. & Ling, W. (1996), Sexual HIV risk and gay and bisexual methamphetamine abusers. *J. Substance Abuse Treatment*, 13(6): 483-386.

Greenwood, G.L., White, E., Page-Shafer, K., Bein, E., Paul, J., Osmond, D. & Stall, R.D. (2000), Correlates of heavy substance use among young gay and bisexual men: The San Francisco young men's health study. *Drug & Alcohol Dependence*, 61:105-112.

Guss, J.R. (2000), Sex like you can't even imagine: "Crystal," crack, and gay men. *J. Gay & Lesbian Psychotherapy*, 3(3/4): 105-122. Reprinted in *Addictions in the Gay and Lesbian Community*, eds. J.R. Guss & J. Drescher. New York: The Haworth Press, Inc., pp. 105-122.

Halkitis, P.N., Fischgrund, B.N. & Parsons, J.T. (2005), Explanations for methamphetamine use among gay and bisexual men in New York City. *Substance Use & Misuse*, 40: 1-5.

Halkitis, P.N., Green, K.A. & Mourgues, P. (2005), Longitudinal investigation of methamphetamine use among gay and bisexual men in New York City: Findings from Project BUMPS. *J. Urban Health*, 82(1, Suppl 1): 18-25.

Halkitis, P.N. & Parsons, J.T. (2002), Recreational drug use and HIV risk sexual behavior among men frequenting urban gay venues. *J. Gay & Lesbian Social Services*, 14(2): 19-38.

Halkitis, P.N., Parsons, J.T. & Stirratt, M. (2001), A double epidemic: Crystal methamphetamine use and its relation to HIV prevention among gay men. *J. Homosexuality*, 41(2): 17-35.

Halkitis, P.N., Parsons, J.T. & Wilton, L. (2003), Characteristics of gay and bisexual
methamphetamine users and contexts of use in New York City. *J. Drug Issues*,
33(2): 413-432.

Halkitis, P.N., Shrem, M.T. & Martin, F.W. (2005), Sexual behavior patterns of methamphetamine using gay and bisexual men in New York City. *Substance Use & Misuse*, 40: 703-709.

Harris, N.V., Thiede, H., McGough, J.P. & Gordon, D. (1993), Risk factors for HIV infection among injecting drug users: Results of blinded surveys in drug treatment
centers, King County, Washington 1988-1991. *J. Acquired Immune Deficiency
Syndromes*, 6(11): 1275-1282.

Mansergh, G., Colfax, G., Marks, G., Rader, M., Guzman, R. & Buchbinder, S. (2001),
The Circuit Party Men's Health Survey: Findings and implications for gay and bisexual men. *American J. Public Health*, 91:953-958.

Mattison, A.M., Ross, M.W., Wolfson, T. & Franklin, D. (2001), Circuit party attendance, club drug use, and unsafe sex in gay men. *J. Substance Abuse*, 13:119-126.

McKirnan, D., Ostrow, D.G. & Hope, B. (1996), Sex, drugs, and escape: A psychological model of HIV-risk sexual behaviors. *AIDS Care*, 8(6): 655-669.

Nemoto, T., Operario, D. & Soma, T. (2002), Risk behaviors of Filipino methamphetamine users in San Francisco: Implications for prevention and treatment of drug use
and HIV. *Public Health Reports*, 117(Supp. 1): S30-38.

New York City Department of Health (2002), New York City HIV/AIDS Surveillance
Statistics 2002. New York: New York City Department of Health and Mental Hygiene, 2004. Posted September 14, 2004. (Accessed at *http://www.nyc.gov/html/
doh/html/ah/hivtables2002.html*).

Parsons, J.T. & Halkitis, P.N. (2002), Sexual and drug using practices of HIV+ men
who frequent public and commercial sex environments. *AIDS Care*, 14: 816-826.

Rawson, R.A., Gonzales, R. & Brethen, P. (2002), Treatment of methamphetamine use
disorders: An update. *J. Substance Abuse Treatment*, 23:145-150.

Reback, C.J. (1997), *The Social Construction of a Gay Drug: Methamphetamine Use
among Gay and Bisexual Males in Los Angeles*. Los Angeles: City of Los Angeles,
AIDS Coordinator's Office.

Semple, S.J., Patterson, T.L & Grant, I. (2002), Motivations associated with methamphetamine use among HIV+ men who have sex with men. *J. Substance Abuse
Treatment*, 22: 149-156.

Shoptaw, S., Reback, C.J. & Freese, T.E. (2002), Patient characteristics, HIV serostatus,
and risk behaviors among gay and bisexual males seeking treatment for methamphetamine abuse and dependence in Los Angeles. *J. Addictive Diseases*, 21:
91-105.

Sorvillo, F., Kerndt, P., Cheng, K., Beall, G., Turner, P.A., Beer, V.L & Kovacs, A.
(1995), Emerging patterns of HIV transmission: The value of alternative surveillance methods. *AIDS*, 9: 625-629.

Vittinghoff, E., Douglas, J., Judson, F., McKirnan, D., MacQueen, K. & Buchbinder, S.P. (1999), Per-contact risk of human immunodeficiency virus transmission between male sexual partners. *American J. Epidemiology*, 150: 1-6.

Woody, G.E., VanEtten-Lee, M.L., McKirnan, D., Donnell, D., Metzger, D., Seage, G. & Gross, M. (2001), Substance use among men who have sex with men: Comparison with a national household survey. *J. Acquired Immune Deficiency Syndrome*, 27: 86-90.

Club Drug Use and Risky Sex Among Gay and Bisexual Men in New York City

José E. Nanín, EdD
Jeffrey T. Parsons, PhD

SUMMARY. In New York City, the use of "club drugs" such as MDMA, crystal methamphetamine, ketamine, GHB, and cocaine has been identified as an emerging problem among subgroups of the gay and bisexual male community. More alarming is the mounting empirical evidence showing how club drug use is associated with the rising prevalence of unsafe sexual behaviors among members of this community, leading to increasing HIV incidence. Studies have been conducted at the Center for HIV Educational Studies and Training (CHEST) at Hunter College of City University of New York that address prevalence of club drug use and unsafe sexual behaviors among various samples of gay and bisexual men in New York City. Creative educational interventions as well as clinical strategies using Motivational Interviewing and Cognitive Behavioral Therapy may be useful for

José E. Nanín and Jeffrey T. Parsons are affiliated with the Center for HIV Educational Studies and Training. Dr. Parsons is also affiliated with Hunter College and the Graduate Center of the City University of New York (CUNY).

Address correspondence to: Jeffrey T. Parsons, PhD, Hunter College-CUNY, Department of Psychology, 695 Park Avenue, New York, NY 10021 (E-mail: Jeffrey.parsons@hunter.cuny.edu).

The authors would like to thank David Bimbi and Elana Rosof for their assistance in preparing this manuscript.

[Haworth co-indexing entry note]: "Club Drug Use and Risky Sex Among Gay and Bisexual Men in New York City." Nanín, José E., and Jeffrey T. Parsons. Co-published simultaneously in *Journal of Gay & Lesbian Psychotherapy* (The Haworth Medical Press, an imprint of The Haworth Press, Inc.) Vol. 10, No. 3/4, 2006, pp. 111-122; and: *Crystal Meth and Men Who Have Sex with Men: What Mental Health Care Professionals Need to Know* (ed: Milton L. Wainberg, Andrew J. Kolodny, and Jack Drescher) The Haworth Medical Press, an imprint of The Haworth Press, Inc., 2006, pp. 111-122. Single or multiple copies of this article are available for a fee from The Haworth Document Delivery Service [1-800-HAWORTH, 9:00 a.m. - 5:00 p.m. (EST). E-mail address: docdelivery@haworthpress.com].

clinicians and other health care practitioners by helping clients develop skills to reduce club drug use and risky sex. *[Article copies available for a fee from The Haworth Document Delivery Service: 1-800-HAWORTH. E-mail address: <docdelivery@haworthpress.com> Website: <http://www.HaworthPress.com>*

KEYWORDS. AIDS, anal intercourse, barebacking, bisexual men, club drugs, cocaine, cognitive-behavioral therapy, crystal meth, gay men, GHB, HIV, homosexuality, ketamine, men having sex with men (MSM), motivational interviewing, risk factors, seroconversion, unsafe sex

A specific set of drugs, known colloquially as "club drugs," has become increasingly available in New York City and other urban areas of the United States (Stall et al., 2001; Klitzman et al., 2002). Along with this rise in availability has come increased demand and use, especially among gay and bisexual men who frequent dance clubs and sex clubs (Halkitis et al., 2001; 2003; Halkitis and Parsons, 2002; Parsons, 2004; Parsons and Halkitis, 2002). This emerging problem poses a threat to the psychological and physical health of gay and bisexual men.

"Club drugs" typically include the following substances: methylene-dioxy-methamphetamine (MDMA or "ecstasy"), crystal methamphetamine, cocaine, ketamine ("K") and gamma-hydroxybutyrate (GHB or "G"). These drugs have been shown to adversely affect memory, attention, and movement and negative psychological side effects are usually reported (Dillon et al., 2001; Topp et al., 1999; Volkow et al., 2001a; 2001b). MDMA use has been shown to cause significant impairments in cognitive functioning, including visual and verbal memory, reasoning, and ability to sustain attention (Curran and Travill, 1997; Rodgers, 2000). Methamphetamine is very addictive and its abuse has been linked to aggressive behavior, paranoia, and potential cardiac and neurological damage (DEA, 2000; NIDA, 2001).

Cocaine, available in most urban areas on the United States, has been linked with such short-term physiological effects as dilated pupils, constricted blood vessels, and increased blood pressure, heart rate, and temperature; yet, high doses or binge use may produce more serious physiological effects. Prolonged use can result in heart disease, respiratory failure, or stroke, and may result in drug-related death (National Institute on Drug Abuse, 1999). Despite these dangerous consequences, some young people view cocaine as a "safer, more predictable alternative to MDMA or amphetamines" (Boys et al., 2001).

Ketamine use disrupts attentional function, explicit memory, and verbal fluency (Adler et al., 1998; Harborne et al., 1996). Schizophrenia-like and dissociative symptoms can also result (Lahti et al., 1995), as well as impairments in semantic and working memory (Adler et al., 1998). GHB, a central nervous system depressant, relaxes and sedates the body. When used with alcohol, which is very likely in a dance club environment, it can result in respiratory depression (LoVecchio et al., 1998). Users of GHB also report adverse effects including dizziness, seizures, nausea, drowsiness, respiratory distress, violent agitation, and amnesia, and can include coma or death (Ingels et al., 2000; Thomas et al., 1997).

Use of a "trail mix," the combination of two or more drugs to achieve desired effects (Halkitis et al., 2003; Parsons et al., 2006), is popular in the gay dance scene (e.g., crushed MDMA, crystal, and ketamine). The term itself implies a casual attitude towards polydrug use (Parsons, 2004). As a result of using multiple drugs, users risk experiencing enhanced negative psychophysiological effects.

CLUB DRUG USE AND HIV SEXUAL RISK

Recreational drug use, in general, places gay and bisexual men at greater risk for HIV seroconversion by increasing the likelihood of unprotected anal intercourse, which has been shown to be the most risky behavior for HIV transmission (Vittinghoff et al., 1999). This is particularly true for club drugs, which have been shown to influence the sexual behaviors of users (Bochow, 1998; Halkitis and Parsons, 2003; Lewis and Ross, 1995; Parsons, 2004). The role of these drugs in facilitating unsafe sexual behaviors among gay/bisexual men has been well documented (CDC 2003a; 2003b; New York City Department of Health and Mental Hygiene, 2004; Valleroy et al., 2000). Among men who have sex with men (MSM) recruited from dance clubs in NYC, MDMA was identified as a risk factor for unprotected anal sex (Klitzman et al., 2000). Although GHB has been marketed as a sexual performance enhancer (Winickoff et al., 2000), and use of the drug has been linked with sexual assault (Slaughter, 2000), it is still not known how much of an effect GHB has on sexual risk practices. In addition, both Mattison and colleagues (2001) and Ross and colleagues (2003) have identified a relationship between ketamine and GHB use and HIV sexual risk among MSM who frequent circuit parties.

Recent studies conducted at the Center for HIV Educational Studies and Training (CHEST) at Hunter College show significant rates of club drug use among members of general gay male populations that may not necessarily frequent dance or sex clubs. The Sex and Love Survey, a brief intercept survey examining issues of sex, love, and health-related issues in the gay, lesbian, bisexual, transgender, and queer communities, was administered in 2002 and 2003 to ethnically diverse samples. In 2002, a sample of 786 single and non-monogamous gay and bisexually identified men, with a mean age of 36, responded to the survey. A good proportion of the sample was represented by men of color (35.1%) and men of HIV-negative (77.9%) and HIV unknown status (10.1%). Regarding past history of club drug use, the majority reported using cocaine (38.5%), followed by MDMA (35%), ketamine (22.8%), crystal methamphetamine (20.5%), and GHB (12.5%). MDMA was reported as the drug most recently used (i.e., with the last 3 months) (12.8%), followed by cocaine (12%), crystal (7.8%), ketamine (6.7%), and GHB (4.5%). There were fewer reports of recent use with unsafe sex, yet those who did report such behavior reported ecstasy use more often (7.9%), followed by cocaine (7.5%), crystal (6.1%), GHB (3.7%), and ketamine (3.7%).

Evidence showing a link between club drug use and HIV sexual risk behaviors was found in this study. Crystal users, regardless of HIV status, were more likely to report recent unprotected anal sex (i.e., within the last 3 months) with men of HIV-negative or unknown status (OR = 3.47, CI = 1.81-6.64, p = 000). HIV-positive men who have unprotected insertive anal sex with partners of HIV-negative or unknown status were more likely to use GHB (OR = 3.56, CI = 1.54-8.18, p = 003) when compared to other club drugs. HIV-negative men having unprotected receptive anal sex with HIV-positive or unknown status partners were more likely to use crystal methamphetamine (OR = 5.06, CI = 2.74-9.37, p = 000). Men who "bareback" (i.e., intentional unprotected sex) were more likely to use stimulants, particularly crystal methamphetamine (OR = 3.08, CI = 1.51-6.31, p = .002) and cocaine (OR = 2.39, CI = 1.19-4.81, p = .01).

Project SPIN, funded by the CDC between 2000 and 2003, included an assessment study of gay/bisexual men who feel that their sexual behaviors are out of control. The aims of the study were to investigate the nature, antecedents, and course of sexual compulsivity (SC) in gay and bisexual men, to evaluate the relationship between SC and HIV sexual risk behaviors, and to determine if SC can be reliably operationalized and distinguished from other disorders using a newly designed diagnostic instrument for SC.

The sample (n = 183) was ethnically diverse, with men of color representing 40.4%. Mean age of participants was 36 (SD = 8.33). The average number of male sexual partners in the prior 3 months was 38.75 (SD = 54.7). Scores on the Kalichman SC scale can range from a low of 10 to a high of 40. The mean score on the Kalichman SC scale for this sample was 31.86 (SD = 4.28).

Prevalence of club drug use among HIV-negative men in this sample (n = 138) included cocaine (25.4%), crystal methamphetamine (19.6%), ecstasy (18.8%), ketamine (15.2%), and GHB (7.2%). Among HIV-positive men, crystal is the most popular club drug (33.3%), followed by cocaine (22.2%), ecstasy (20.0%), ketamine (13.3%), and GHB (11.1%). The study also assessed use of amyl nitrate ("poppers") and Viagra (silfenadil) (regardless of prescription status) because of their popularity among gay men for use in dance clubs and during sexual activity. Poppers were highly used among both HIV-negative (42%) and HIV-positive men (51.1%). Viagra was used among 25.4% of the HIV-negative men and 40% of the HIV-positive men.

In comparison to the Sex and Love sample, the SPIN participants reported 50% to 300% more club drug use. The largest disparity was in crystal methamphetamine use (7.8% vs. 23%). However, this may be due to the nature of the study (i.e., being sexually out of control, which many participants linked to their use of crystal methamphetamine).

More SPIN participants also reported lifetime history of STIs. In SPIN, 60.1% of the HIV-negative men reported having STIs compared to 35.2% of the HIV-negative men in Sex and Love. Over eighty percent of HIV-positive men in SPIN (84.4%) reported this compared to 73.3% of HIV-positive men in Sex and Love.

More SPIN participants also identified as "barebackers," men who have intentional anal sex without condoms. Of the HIV-negative men in SPIN, 14.6% identified as such compared to 8.9 % of HIV-negative men in Sex and Love. Similarly, 40% of HIV-positive men in SPIN reported being a "barebacker" compared to 33.7% HIV-positive men in Sex and Love.

In summary, Project SPIN contained a sample of men with a wide-ranging repertoire of sex-related problem behaviors including club drug use, compared to other samples of gay/bisexual men from New York City. Higher rates of HIV sexual risk behaviors, higher rates of past STIs, increased use of club drugs, several significant differences between HIV+ and HIV-men, increased use of methamphetamine and Viagra, higher rates of past STIs, and higher likelihood to identify as a "barebacker" (Parsons, Morgenstern and Bimbi, 2004).

The Sex and Love Survey showed rates of club drug use in the past 3 months ranging from 12.8% to 4.5%. Both HIV-positive and HIV-negative men who reported serodiscordant unprotected sex were more likely to be club drug users. In accordance with results from other studies (e.g., Mansergh et al., 2001; Mattison et al., 2001; Ross et al., 2003), Sex and Love also has shown a clear relationship between sexual risk (including barebacking) and club drug use (Parsons and Halkitis, 2003). Project SPIN has documented the importance of looking at the unique intersection of sexual compulsivity, sexual risk behaviors, and club drug use. Significant clinical intervention implications are thus implied.

FOCUS ON CRYSTAL METHAMPHETAMINE USE

The first several months of 2004 saw increasing attention to the "epidemic" of crystal methamphetamine among gay/bisexual men in New York City. Several articles appeared in the mainstream and gay press, alerting readers to this new health issue (see Jacobs, 2004; Kaiser Family Foundation, 2004; Osborne, 2004). The rise of crystal methamphetamine use and high risk sex among gay/bisexual men in New York City is now being identified as a significant problem for gay men to deal with as well as for their health care providers.

This newfound attention is warranted, considering the adverse impact crystal methamphetamine is having on the health of members of the gay male community. A study conducted in 1998 by Halkitis and Parsons (2002) revealed that 9.9% reported crystal methamphetamine use in the prior three months. Interestingly, most of these men were using crystal methamphetamine less than once a month. Another study conducted between 1997-1998 (Purcell et al., 2001) revealed that, out of a sample of 456 HIV-positive men (from NYC and SF), 11.6% reported any amphetamine use (including crystal methamphetamine) in the prior 3 months. Methamphetamine users reported significantly more acts of unprotected receptive anal sex with HIV-negative or unknown status partners. Another study conducted with young adults aged 18-25 in New York City in 2001 revealed that 14.3% of the gay/bisexual males in the sample had used crystal methamphetamine in the prior 6 months (Parsons, Halkitis and Bimbi, 2006).

The Seropositive Urban Men's Intervention Trial (SUMIT), a CDC-funded project, conducted between 2000-2001 was a randomized intervention for HIV-positive, ethnically-diverse gay/bisexual men in New York City and San Francisco. In this study, 10.7% of the sample had used crystal in the 3 months prior to their first interview. Methamphetamine users were twice as likely to report unprotected anal sex with HIV-negative and unknown status casual partners (Purcell et al., 2005).

In the Sex and Love Survey, comparison of the data from participants recruited in 2002 and those recruited in 2003 revealed no significant difference in reporting *ever* using crystal (20.5% in 2002 and 19.9% in 2003). However, there was a significant increase in *recent* use (last 3 months): from 7.8% in 2003 to 10.6% in 2003.

Considering the increase in crystal methamphetamine use over the past few years, the number of CMA groups and those presenting with methamphetamine dependence has increased. This creates a burden on clinical practitioners and other health and social service providers to enhance or create services in response to this emerging "epidemic."

INTERVENTION IMPLICATIONS: PSYCHOEDUCATION

The substantial qualitative and quantitative formative research with gay and bisexual men conducted at CHEST has consistently shown that gay and bisexual male club drug users do not want to be lectured to, nor are they always interested in support groups. They do seem to respond to humorous, entertaining approaches to safer sex and other health education. An example of this is the Drag Initiative to Vanquish AIDS (DIVA), a group of gay men involved in HIV research and education who dress up in wigs and costumes (Parsons, 2004). Recently, DIVA has been involved with club promoters and the New York City Department of Health and Mental Hygiene in outreach efforts to encourage gay and bisexual men, including club drug users, to get tested for HIV and other STIs and to receive other important health services (e.g., smoking cessation products, mental health screening).

Another intervention developed in response to this need was the creation of a video entitled "The Biggest Mess." This is an "edu-tainment" video that provides factual information about drug use, physical and psychological effects, impact on immune system (for HIV-positive men in particular), and relationship to sexual risk behaviors among gay/bisexual men, but the information is presented in a campy, comedic, and entertaining manner. The video can be used within a club or bar setting to entertain and educate patrons of such venues. It can also be used in medical and social service settings catering to gay and bisexual men, as a waiting room video or as part of an educational workshop or individual session.

Although not empirically validated, the response from select groups of viewers has been very positive, rating it as engaging, informative, accurate, and fun. It is currently being used in a research project at CHEST and in other programs across the United States, the United Kingdom, Europe, and Australia.

INTERVENTION IMPLICATIONS: PSYCHOLOGICAL COUNSELING

As previously mentioned, gay and bisexual club drug users in past studies at CHEST expressed desire for educational programs that provide facts without being "preachy" or "boring." DIVA outreach and "The Biggest Mess" video are only two examples out of many that exist. Yet, based on information from CHEST studies, men who are more concerned about their club drug use are interested in individual-level counseling. These men require access to effective counseling services to assist them with their drug use and other related issues.

Much cause for concern among clinicians and other health care and social service providers has been raised throughout this article. It is even more imperative for providers to have the information and tools necessary to offer culturally-appropriate and non-judgmental services for gay and bisexual men who want to reduce and/or cease their use of club drugs and rediscover the benefits of safer sex.

Providers may adopt skills in Motivational Interviewing (Miller and Rollnick, 1991, 2002) and Cognitive Behavioral Therapy (CBT) to ease this process. As reported in other articles in this volume (Bux and Irwin, 2006; Irwin, 2006), MI and CBT are highly recommended counseling modalities for facilitating change in behavior among gay/bisexual male club drug users. MI is an effective approach for practitioners and other service providers to use with gay and bisexual men because of its non-judgmental orientation and integration with harm reduction strategies (Parsons, 2004). CBT is extremely useful because it helps clients develop skills in avoiding risky situations and managing their recovery despite environments with many triggers to use again. Currently, we are involved with a NIDA-funded behavioral intervention, in conjunction with our colleagues at Columbia University, called Project PnP ("Party-n-Play"),[1] which is currently being evaluated to use four MI sessions to reduce risky sex and club drug use among gay/bi men.

CONCLUSION

The information provided in this article was provided to inform and encourage further research and intervention development for clinicians and other providers who seek to assist gay and bisexual men with reducing or ceasing club drug use and practicing healthier sexual behaviors. Adopting the educational and counseling strategies mentioned in this paper and throughout this journal, as well as other effective prevention and treatment strategies discussed in other sources, is highly encouraged. In doing so, clinicians will be furthering the cause of helping members of our gay and bisexual community avoid another health crisis.

NOTE

1. "Party-n-Play" is the colloquial term used by gay and bisexual men to describe drug use before and during sexual activity (Hirshfield et al., 2004).

REFERENCES

Adler, C.M., Goldberg, T.E., Malhotra, A.K., Pickar, D. & Breier, A. (1998), Effects of ketamine on thought disorder, working memory, and semantic memory in health volunteers. *Biological Psychiatry*, 43:811-816.

Bochow, M. (1998), The importance of contextualizing research: An analysis of data from the German gay press survey. *J. Psychology & Human Sexuality*, 10:37-58.

Bux, D. & Irwin, T. (2006), Combining motivational interviewing and cognitive-behavioral therapy for the treatment of crystal methamphetamine abuse/dependence. *J. Gay & Lesbian Psychotherapy*, 10(3/4): 143-152.

Centers for Disease Control and Prevention (CDC) (2003a), *Press Release: New Study Shows Overall Increase in HIV Diagnoses*. Office of Communications, November 26, 2003.

Centers for Disease Control and Prevention (CDC) (2003b). Press Release: *HIV Diagnoses Climbing Among Gay and Bisexual Men*. Office of Communications, July 28, 2003.

Curran, H.V. & Travill, R.A. (1997), Mood and cognitive effects of 3,4,-methylenedioxymethamphetamine (MDMA, 'ecstasy'): Weekend "high" followed by midweek "low." *Addiction*, 92(7):821-831.

Dillon, P., Copeland, J. & Jansen, K. (2001), *Patterns of Use and Harms Associated with Non-medical Ketamine Use*. New South Wales, Australia: National Drug and Alcohol Research Centre. NDARC Technical Report No. 111.

Drug Enforcement Administration (DEA) (2000), *An Overview of Club Drugs*. Washington, DC: Drug Intelligence Brief, February.

Halkitis, P.N. & Parsons, J.T. (2002), Recreational drug use and HIV-risk sexual be-havior among men frequenting gay social venues. *J. Gay & Lesbian Social Services*, 14:19-39.

Halkitis, P.N. & Parsons, J.T. (2003), Intentional unsafe sex (barebacking) among HIV Seropositive gay men who seek sexual partners on the Internet. *AIDS Care*, 15:367-378.

Halkitis, P.N., Parsons, J.T. & Stirratt, M. (2001), A double epidemic: Crystal metham-phetamine use and its relation to HIV transmission among gay men. *J. Homosexuality*, 41:17-35.

Halkitis, P.N., Parsons, J.T. & Wilton, L. (2003), An exploratory study of contextual and situational factors related to methamphetamine use among gay and bisexual men in New York City. *J. Drug Issues*, 33:413-432.

Hirshfield, S., Remien, R.H., Humberstone, M., Walavalkar, I. & Chiasson, M.A. (2004), Substance use and high-risk sex among men who have sex with men: a na-tional online study in the USA. *AIDS Care*, 16:1036-1047.

Ingels, M., Rangan, C., Bellezzo, J. & Clark, R.F. (2000), Coma and respiratory de-pression following the ingestion of GHB and its precursors: Three cases. *J. Emer-gency Medicine*, 19:47-50.

Irwin, T. (2006), Strategies for the treatment of methamphetamine use disorders among gay and bisexual men. *J. Gay & Lesbian Psychotherapy*, 10(3/4): 131-141.

Jacobs, A. (2004), The beast in the bathhouse: Crystal meth use by gay men threatens to reignite an epidemic. *New York Times*, January 12; Sect. B:1 (col. 2).

Kaiser Family Foundation (2004), New York City health workers say crystal meth use helping to spread HIV among men who have sex with men. *Kaiser Daily HIV/AIDS Report*, January 12.

Klitzman, R.L., Greenberg, J.D., Pollack, L.M. & Dolezal, C. (2002), MDMA ("ec-stasy") use, and its association with high risk behaviors, mental health, and other factors among gay/bisexual men in New York City. *Drug & Alcohol Dependence*, 66:115-125.

Klitzman, R.L., Pope, H.G., Jr. & Hudson, J.I. (2000), MDMA ("Ecstasy") abuse and high-risk sexual behaviors among 169 gay and bisexual men. *American J. Psychia-try*, 157:1162-1164.

Lahti, A.C., Holcomb, H.H., Medoff, D.R. & Tamminga, C.A. (1995), Ketamine acti-vates psychosis and alters limbic blood flow in schizophrenia. *Neuroreport*, 6:869-872.

Lewis, L.A. & Ross, M.W. (1995), The gay dance party culture in Sydney: A qualita-tive analysis. *J. Homosexuality*, 29:41-70.

Mansergh, G., Colfax, G., Marks, G., Rader, M., Guzman, R. & Buchbinder, S. (2001), The Circuit Party Men's Health Survey: Findings and implications for gay and bi-sexual men. *American J. Public Health*, 91:953-958.

Mattison, A.M., Ross, M.W., Wolfson, T. & Franklin, D. (2001), Circuit party atten-dance, club drug use, and unsafe sex in gay men. *J. Substance Abuse*, 13:119-126.

Miller, W.R. & Rollnick, S. (1991), *Motivational Interviewing: Preparing People to Change*. New York: Guilford Press.

Miller, W.R. & Rollnick, S. (2002), *Motivational Interviewing: Preparing People to Change. (2nd ed.)*. New York: Guilford Press.

National Institute on Drug Abuse (NIDA) (1999), *Cocaine Abuse and Addiction.* Bethesda: U.S. Department of Health and Human Services. NIDA Research Report Series, Publication #99-4342, May.

National Institute on Drug Abuse (NIDA) (2001), *Methamphetamine.* Bethesda: U.S. Department of Health and Human Services. NIDA Infofax.

New York City Department of Health and Mental Hygiene (2004), Health Bulletin: Methamphetamine and HIV. *Health & Mental Hygiene News,* 3(3).

Osborne, D. (2004), Fight against crystal demanded. *Gay City News,* 3(308), February 19, Available at: http://gaycitynews.com/gcn_308/fightagaintscrystal.html. Accessed February 25, 2004.

Parsons, J.T. (2004), HIV-positive gay and bisexual men. In: *Positive Prevention: Reducing HIV Transmission Among People Living with HIV/AIDS,* ed. S.C. Kalichman. New York: Kluwer, pp. 99-133.

Parsons, J.T. & Halkitis, P.N. (2002), Sexual and drug using practices of HIV+ men who frequent commercial and public sex environments. *AIDS Care,* 14:815-826.

Parsons, J.T. & Halkitis, P.N. (2003), *Club Drug Use and Sexual Risk Behaviors Among Gay/Bisexual Men.* Paper presented at the 131st American Public Health Association annual meeting: San Francisco, CA, Nov.

Parsons, J.T., Halkitis, P.N. & Bimbi, D. (2006), Club drug use among young adults frequenting dance clubs and other social venues in New York City. *J. Child & Adolescent Substance Abuse,* 15(3): 1-14.

Parsons, J.T., Morgenstern, J. & Bimbi, D.S. (2004), *The Role of Sexually Compulsive Symptoms on HIV Sexual Risk Practices and Use of Illicit Drugs Before Sex.* Paper presented at the 15th World AIDS Conference: Bangkok, Thailand, July.

Purcell, D.W., Moss, S., Remien, R.H., Parsons, J.T. & Woods, W.J. (2005), Illicit substance use as a predictor of sexual risk taking behavior among HIV-seropositive gay and bisexual men. *AIDS,* 19(S1): 537-547.

Purcell, D.W., Parsons, J.T., Halkitis, P.N., Mizuno, Y. & Woods, W. (2001), Relationship of substance use by HIV-seropositive men who have sex with men and unprotected anal intercourse with HIV-negative and unknown serostatus partners. *J. Substance Abuse,* 13(1-2):185-200

Rodgers, J. (2000), Cognitive performance amongst recreational users of "ecstasy." *Psychopharmacology,* 151:19-24.

Ross, M., Mattison, A. & Franlin, D. (2003), Club drugs and sex on drugs are associated with different motivations for gay circuit party attendance in men. *Substance Use & Misuse,* 38:1171-1179.

Slaughter, J. (2000), Beyond outrage. *Revolution,* 1:28-35.

Stall, R., Paul, J.P., Greenwood, G., Pollack, L. M., Bein, E., Crosby, G.M., Mills, T.C., Binson, D., Coates, T.J. & Catania, J.A. (2001), Alcohol use, drug use and alcohol-related problems among men who have sex with men: The Urban Men's Health Study, *Addiction,* 96:1589-1601.

Thomas, G., Bonner, S. & Gascoigne, A. (1997), Coma induced by abuse of hydroxybutyrate (GBH or liquid ecstasy): A case report. *Bio Medical Journal,* 314:35.

Topp, L., Hando, J., Dillon, P., Roche, A. & Solowij, N. (1999), Ecstasy use in Australia: Patterns of use associated with harm. *Drug & Alcohol Dependency,* 55:105-115.

Valleroy, L.A., Mackellar, D.A., Karon, J.M., Daniel, H., McFarland, W., Shehan, D.A., et al. (2000), HIV prevalence and associated risks in young men who have sex with men. *J. American Medical Association*, 284:198-204.

Vittinghoff, E., Douglas, J., Judson, F., McKirnan, D., MacQueen, K. & Buchbinger, S.P. (1999), Per-contact risk of Human Immunodeficiency Virus transmission between male sexual partners. *American J. Epidemiology*, 150:1-6.

Volkow, N.D., Chang, L., Wang, G.J., Fowler, J.S., Franceschi, D., Sedler, M.J., et al. (2001a), Higher cortical and lower subcortical metabolism in detoxified methamphetamine abusers. *American J. Psychiatry*, 158:383-389.

Volkow, N.D., Chang, L., Wang, G.J., Fowler, J.S., Leonido-Yee, M., Franceschi, D., et al. (2001b), Association of dopamine transporter reduction with psychomotor impairment in methamphetamine abusers. *American J. Psychiatry*, 158:377-383.

Winickoff, J.P., Houck, C.S., Rothman, E.L. & Bauchner, H. (2000), Verve and jolt: Deadly new internet drugs. *Pediatrics*, 106:829-831.

HIV Risk Behaviors Among Gay Male Methamphetamine Users: Before and After Treatment

Sherry Larkins, PhD
Cathy J. Reback, PhD
Steven Shoptaw, PhD

SUMMARY. Methamphetamine-using gay men are at high risk for HIV transmission, largely due to the high-risk sexual risk behaviors they engage in while using the drug. Gay men who use the drug frequently report that it enables them to have intense, long-lasting sexual encounters. Substance abuse treatment interventions that target both substance use and sexual behavior have been successful in helping gay men reduce their

---

Sherry Larkins is affiliated with the University of California, Los Angeles, Integrated Substance Abuse Programs (UCLA ISAP), Los Angeles, CA.

Cathy J. Reback is affiliated with the University of California, Los Angeles, Integrated Substance Abuse Programs (UCLA ISAP), Los Angeles, CA; Friends Research Institute, Inc., Los Angeles, CA; and Van Ness Recovery House, Los Angeles, CA.

Steven Shoptaw is affiliated with the University of California, Los Angeles, Integrated Substance Abuse Programs (UCLA ISAP), Los Angeles, CA; University of California, Los Angeles, Center for HIV Identification, Prevention and Treatment Services (CHIPTS); and Friends Research Institute, Inc., Los Angeles, CA.

Address correspondence to: Sherry Larkins, PhD, UCLA ISAP, 11075 Santa Monica Boulevard, Suite #200, Los Angeles, CA 90025 (E-mail: slarkins@mindspring. com).

[Haworth co-indexing entry note]: "HIV Risk Behaviors Among Gay Male Methamphetamine Users: Before and After Treatment." Larkins, Sherry, Cathy J. Reback, and Steven Shoptaw. Co-published simultaneously in *Journal of Gay & Lesbian Psychotherapy* (The Haworth Medical Press, an imprint of The Haworth Press, Inc.) Vol. 10, No. 3/4, 2006, pp. 123-129; and: *Crystal Meth and Men Who Have Sex with Men: What Mental Health Care Professionals Need to Know* (ed: Milton L. Wainberg, Andrew J. Kolodny, and Jack Drescher) The Haworth Medical Press, an imprint of The Haworth Press, Inc., 2006, pp. 123-129. Single or multiple copies of this article are available for a fee from The Haworth Document Delivery Service [1-800-HAWORTH, 9:00 a.m. - 5:00 p.m. (EST). E-mail address: docdelivery@haworthpress.com].

Available online at http://jglp.haworthpress.com
doi:10.1300/J236v10n03_11

sexual risks including: reducing the number of sexual partners, reducing the frequency of unprotected anal intercourse, and reducing frequency of public sex encounters. Such treatments have the potential to curtail the spread of HIV and other sexually-transmitted infections (STIs), while simultaneously treating the substance abuse disorder. *[Article copies available for a fee from The Haworth Document Delivery Service: 1-800-HAWORTH. E-mail address: <docdelivery@haworthpress.com> Website: <http://www.HaworthPress.com> © 2006 by The Haworth Press, Inc. All rights reserved.]*

KEYWORDS. AIDS, anal intercourse, gay men, HIV, homosexuality, men having sex with men (MSM), methamphetamine, risk reduction, sexual risk, STI, substance abuse

INTRODUCTION

A variety of data sources suggest that methamphetamine use has been increasing in the United States over the last decade (Arrestee Drug Abuse Monitoring Program, 2003; Drug Abuse Warning Network, 2001; National Institute on Drug Abuse, 2001). It has been particularly popular among some sub-populations, including gay men (Gorman 1997; Semple, Patterson and Grant, 2002). This potent stimulant has been closely related to sexual expression and experiences among gay men living in urban centers on the west coast (e.g., Los Angeles, San Francisco) (Mansergh et al., 2001; Molitor et al., 1998; Reback, 1997) and evidence suggests its influence is moving to midwestern and east coast cities as well (Colfax et al., 2004; Halkitis, Parsons and Wilton, 2003; McNall and Remafedi, 1999; Woody et al., 2001).

Methamphetamine's devastating effect on the sexual health of gay men has been of great public concern. Use of the drug has been associated with several sexual risk factors including decreased condom use (Purcell et al., 2001), decreased HIV disclosure among sexual partners (Larkins, Reback and Shoptaw, 2005), increased number of sexual partners (Molitor et al., 1998; Reback, Larkins and Shoptaw, 2004), and increased likelihood of engaging in anal sex (Reback, Larkins and Shoptaw, 2004). Not surprisingly, use of methamphetamine among gay men is also associated with increased rates of HIV infection (Chesney, Barrett and Stall, 1998). As a result, significant prevention and treatment efforts have recently been put forth to address these public health concerns.

In the last decade, several social marketing campaigns were designed to discourage methamphetamine use among gay men; they highlighted the disturbing connection between the drug's use and HIV infection (e.g., NYC's "Buy Crystal, get HIV Free!;" Miami's "METH = DEATH."). In addition to these prevention efforts, there have also been substance abuse treatment interventions specifically targeting gay men. Such interventions have integrated material on sexual identity, sexuality, and intimacy into their curricula. These interventions have focused on the role of methamphetamine in the sexual and social lives of gay men, and how individuals can develop tools for stopping use, preventing relapse, and preventing the high-risk sex often associated with the use of the drug.

This paper discusses the benefits of a substance abuse treatment intervention that targeted gay men. We argue that addressing both the methamphetamine use and its associated high-risk sex are of paramount importance when treating an addiction that is so intertwined with sexual behavior. Gay-targeted treatment interventions that address drug use as well as sex and intimacy have the benefit of confronting high-risk sex and helping individuals to develop skills for preventing relapses to both drug use and high-risk sex. Such interventions can potentially prevent further spread of HIV and other sexually-transmitted infections (STIs). Data from one study evaluating a gay-targeted intervention suggests that receiving treatment for methamphetamine use can significantly reduce individuals' sexual risks during treatment (Shoptaw et al., 2005).

THE METHAMPHETAMINE-SEX CONNECTION AMONG GAY MEN ENROLLED IN TREATMENT

Over the last several years, our research group (UCLA ISAP) has provided treatment to methamphetamine-dependent gay men throughout southern California. Consistently, we have seen a very large number (80+%) report that methamphetamine and sexual activities "always" or "often" go together. Comments participants make about methamphetamine are that it makes sexual encounters "intense," "long-lasting," "uninhibited," "kinky," "heightened," and "wild" (Reback, Larkins and Shoptaw, 2004). Many participants comment on the sexual benefits methamphetamine brings to an encounter, at least in early stages of use. They speak of their ability to meet people more easily, connect socially and sexually with others, assert their sexual desires, and shed self-consciousness.

However, a significant number of participants (75+%) report that their sexual behaviors become "compulsive" while using the drug, and that the sexual benefits the drug provides are short lived. Many come to view their sexual behavior as "dark," "repetitive," "compulsive," "obsessive," and "risky," and argue that the compulsive nature of their sexual behavior while using the drug contributes to sexual risk-taking (Reback, Larkins and Shoptaw, 2004). For many, methamphetamine usage and sex have become fused; these men believe they will be unable to achieve a satisfying sexual life if they abstain from methamphetamine. Many are apprehensive about initiating sexual contact following a period of sobriety, fearing sex while sober will be awkward, mundane, or unpleasant. This anxiety around sexual performance and pleasure leaves many vulnerable to relapse once abstinence has been achieved.

OUTCOMES FROM A GAY-TARGETED TREATMENT INTERVENTION

The intense relationship between methamphetamine and sexual behavior calls for a treatment approach that addresses both drug use and sexual risk. Almost a decade ago, our group began developing treatment interventions that target gay men whose substance use is entangled with their sexual risk. In one intervention, gay male methamphetamine users enrolled in a 4-month, structured, out-patient research-treatment program where we compared drug use and sexual risk outcomes of: (1) a standard cognitive-behavioral intervention (CBT) that taught thought-stopping, craving management, and relapse analysis skills, with (2) a gay-targeted intervention that integrated core concepts from the standard CBT intervention with relevant behavioral and cultural aspects of methamphetamine use by gay men.

The gay-targeted intervention equally addressed drug abuse treatment and reductions in HIV-related sexual risk behaviors. Experts on the target community worked with the authors on development of the intervention to ensure a culturally relevant approach. Treatment sessions incorporated gay referents. For example, a standard CBT session on trigger identification was modified to help participants identify gay cultural events (e.g., circuit parties, gay pride celebrations) and environments (e.g., sex clubs) that can trigger methamphetamine use. Some sessions encouraged participants to discuss such topics as the types of sexual behaviors they engage in when using and not using the drug, and the parallels between coming out and revealing one's drug problem. Outcomes from this research-treatment trial (N = 162) suggested that participants receiving gay-targeted treatment significantly reduced their high-risk sexual behaviors during treatment more than those men receiving a standard CBT intervention (Shoptaw et al., 2005).

Outcomes From One-Year Follow-Up

Outcomes from a qualitative sub-study (n = 34) of these same men showed that a year following treatment, sexual risk reductions were realized primarily in: (1) the number of monthly sexual partners; (2) the incidence of unprotected anal intercourse; and (3) the incidence of public sex encounters. While the sample was too small to ascertain an intervention effect at one-year follow-up, there was an overall treatment effect showing that participants reduced their sexual risks throughout treatment, and maintained these reductions to 12 months.

At treatment entry (baseline), participants reported an average of 10 unique sexual partners in the previous month. More than 60% reported engaging in unprotected anal sex during in the previous month, and more than half report engaging in sex in public locations (e.g., bathhouse, sex club, public restroom) during the same period. Twelve months following treatment entry, participants reported approximately 3 unique sexual partners in the previous month, a more than 3-fold reduction from baseline. Approximately one-third reported engaging in unprotected anal sex during in the previous month, an almost two-fold reduction from baseline. About one-fifth reported engaging in sex in a public location in the previous month, a more than two-fold reduction between baseline and 12-month follow-up. Thus, following substance abuse treatment, participants not only reduced their substance use (see Reback, Larkins and Shoptaw, 2004), but they reduced the sexual risk behaviors that accompany the drug use as well.

SUBSTANCE ABUSE TREATMENT AS HIV PREVENTION

Substance abuse treatments that address the intersection of methamphetamine use and sexual behavior have the potential to curb the spread of HIV and other STIs, while simultaneously treating the substance abuse disorder. Research has long shown that individuals who are using substances make different decision regarding sexual risk than do those who are not using substances. Our own research (Reback, Larkins and Shoptaw, 2004) has similarly shown that as participants reduce or eliminate their use of methamphetamine, their sexual behaviors change dramatically. We detail this transformation as participants move from actively using substances, through the treatment process, and to one-year post-admission. Substance abuse treatment was shown to help participants break the intimate relationship between methamphetamine and sex. We argue that treatment interventions targeting gay men should confront issues of sexual behavior and help participants develop tools for integrating intimacy back into their lives. Given the widespread fears many methamphetamine-dependent gay men have about engaging in sexual activities while sober, treatment approaches that confront and address issues of intimacy and performance, as well as issues of risk, are vital to the health of gay men.

REFERENCES

Arrestee Drug Abuse Monitoring (ADAM): Annual Report 2000 (April 2003), National Institute of Justice.

Chesney, M.A., Barrett, D.C. & Stall, R. (1998), Histories of substance use and risk behavior precursors to seroconversion in homosexual men. *American J. Public Health*, 88: 113-116.

Colfax, G., Vittinghoff, E., Husnik, M.J., McKirnan, D., Buchbinder, S., Koblin, B., Celum, C., Chesney, M., Huang, Y., Mayer, K., Bozeman, S., Judson, F.N., Bryant, K.J. & Coates, T.J. (2004), Substance use and sexual risk: A participant and episode-level analysis among a cohort of men who have sex with men. *American J. Epidemiology*, 159: 1002-1012.

Drug Abuse Warning Network (2001), Emergency Department Trends from the Drug Abuse Warning Network, Preliminary Estimates January-June 2001 with Revised estimates 1994 to 2000. DAWN Series D-20, Substance Abuse and Mental Health Services Administration, Office of Applied Studies. DHHS Publication No. (SMA) 02-3634. Rockville, MD.

Gorman, E.M., Barr, A.H., Robertson, B. & Green, C. (1997), Speed, sex, gay men, and HIV: Ecological and community perspectives. *Medical Anthropology Quarterly*, 11: 505-515.

Halkitis, P.N., Parsons, J.T. & Wilton, L. (2003), An exploratory study of contextual and situational factors related to methamphetamine use among gay and bisexual men in New York City. *J. Drug Issues*, 33: 413-432.

Larkins, S., Reback, C.J. & Shoptaw, S. (2005), Methamphetamine-dependent gay men's disclosure of their HIV status to sexual partners. *AIDS Care*, 17(4): 521-532.

Mansergh, G., Colfax, G., Marks, G., Rader, M., Guzman, R. & Buchbinder, S. (2001), The Circuit Party Men's Health Survey: Findings and implications for gay and bisexual men. *American J. Public Health*, 91: 953-958.

McNall, M. & Remafedi, G. (1999), Relationship of amphetamine and other substance use to unprotected intercourse among men who have sex with men. *Archives of Pediatric Adolescent Medicine*, 153: 1130-1135.

Molitor, F., Traux, S.R., Ruiz, J.D. & Sun, R.K. (1998), Association of methamphetamine use during sex with risky sexual behaviors and HIV infection among non-injection drug users. *Western J. Medicine*, 168: 93-97.

National Institute on Drug Abuse (2001), CEWG Epidemiologic Trends in Drug Abuse. National Institute on Drug Abuse, Division of Epidemiology, Services, and Prevention Research, National Institute on Drug Abuse, Proceedings of the Community Epidemiology Work Group.

Purcell, D.W., Parsons, J.T., Halkitis, P.N., Mizuno, Y. & Woods, W.J. (2001), Substance use and sexual transmission risk behavior of HIV-positive men who have sex with men. *J. Substance Abuse*, 13: 185-200.

Reback, C.J. (1997), The social construction of a gay drug: Methamphetamine use among gay and bisexual males in Los Angeles. Los Angeles: City of Los Angeles, AIDS Coordinator's Office.

Reback, C.J., Larkins, S. & Shoptaw, S. (2004), Changes in the meaning of sexual risk behaviors among gay and bisexual male methamphetamine abusers before and after drug treatment, *AIDS & Behavior*, 8(1): 87-98.

Semple, S.J., Patterson, T.L. & Grant, I. (2002), Motivations associated with methamphetamine use among HIV+ men who have sex with men. *J. Substance Abuse Treatment*, 22: 149-156.

Shoptaw, S., Reback, C.J., Peck, J., Yang, X., Rotheram-Fuller, E., Larkins, S., Veniegas, R., Freese, T.E. & Hucks-Ortiz. (2005), Behavioral treatment approaches for methamphetamine dependence and HIV-related sexual risk behaviors among urban gay and bisexual men. *Drug & Alcohol Dependence*, 78: 125-134.

Woody, G. E., Van Etten-Lee, M.L., McKirnan, D., Donnell, D., Metzger, D., Seage, G. & Gross, M. (2001), Substance use among men who have sex with men: Comparison with a national household survey. *J. Acquired Immune Deficiency Syndromes*, 27(1): 86-90.

Strategies for the Treatment of Methamphetamine Use Disorders Among Gay and Bisexual Men

Thomas W. Irwin, PhD

SUMMARY. There is a growing need for treatment services that specifically target methamphetamine for gay and bisexual men. There may be significant barriers for the client in engaging in a treatment program, including thought disturbances and paranoia. A high level of ambivalence in spite of extreme adverse consequences from use is also relatively common among those presenting for treatment. Many people do recover if they are willing to commit to a structured treatment plan. Models of treatment that have been shown to be successful include motivational interviewing (MI), cognitive behavioral therapy (CBT), and community reinforcement with contingency management. The Matrix Model was developed specifically for stimulant use disorders and includes many of these components as well as 12-step facilitation. Although it has been suggested that methamphetamine dependence may be more difficult to treat than other drug use dependence, empirical evidence suggests that success for methamphetamine treatment has not been shown to be different than for other stimulants, such as cocaine. *[Article copies available for a fee from The Haworth Document Delivery Service: 1-800-HAWORTH. E-mail address: <docdelivery@haworthpress.com> Website: <http://www.HaworthPress.com> © 2006 by The Haworth Press, Inc. All rights reserved.]*

Thomas W. Irwin is Assistant Professor, Columbia University School of Medicine.

[Haworth co-indexing entry note]: "Strategies for the Treatment of Methamphetamine Use Disorders Among Gay and Bisexual Men." Irwin, Thomas W. Co-published simultaneously in *Journal of Gay & Lesbian Psychotherapy* (The Haworth Medical Press, an imprint of The Haworth Press, Inc.) Vol. 10, No. 3/4, 2006, pp. 131-141; and: *Crystal Meth and Men Who Have Sex with Men: What Mental Health Care Professionals Need to Know* (ed: Milton L. Wainberg, Andrew J. Kolodny, and Jack Drescher) The Haworth Medical Press, an imprint of The Haworth Press, Inc., 2006, pp. 131-141. Single or multiple copies of this article are available for a fee from The Haworth Document Delivery Service [1-800-HAWORTH, 9:00 a.m. - 5:00 p.m. (EST). E-mail address: docdelivery@haworthpress.com].

Available online at http://jglp.haworthpress.com
doi:10.1300/J236v10n03_12

KEYWORDS. Bisexual men, cognitive-behavioral therapy (CBT), gay men, homosexuality, matrix model, men who have sex with men (MSM), methamphetamine, motivational interviewing (MI), substance abuse treatment

METHAMPHETAMINE IN AN ENVIRONMENTAL CONTEXT

An important component of successfully treating methamphetamine (MA) use disorders is understanding the environmental context in which use occurs. One of the challenges that clinicians face is that the environments and ways in which gay and bisexual men use MA are constantly changing. In a relatively short period of time, MA use among gay and bi men in the New York City area has doubled, with estimated use between 10 and 20 percent (Halkitis, Parsons and Stirratt, 2001). Methamphetamine has become an integral part of many of the venues where gay and bi men socialize, such as circuit parties, dance clubs, and bars (Colfax et al., 2001; Mansergh et al., 2001; Reback, 1997), and it has become the drug of choice at these venues because it allows users to participate continuously without need for sleep. However, MA use is not limited to these settings; it is being used by an increasingly diverse group of gay and bisexual men.

Of growing concern to public health officials is the fact that men who have sex with men (MSM) are increasingly using the Internet for the purposes of obtaining access to drugs and sex (Fernandez, 2004). There is research showing that MSM who meet partners on the Internet have higher rates of MA use and have more unprotected sex (Benotsch et al., 2001). The Internet provides an anonymous and efficient vehicle for identifying potential partners who use MA and setting up sexual encounters where the drug is likely to be included. There is no "down time" in these networks and, in urban areas where there is a sufficient density of gay and bisexual men, a man can probably find a sex partner and methamphetamine twenty-four hours a day.

CLINICAL BARRIERS TO TREATMENT

Methamphetamine users are a difficult patient population to treat. There are several reasons why treatment may be difficult. For example, long-term MA users often present with severe psychiatric symptoms (van Gorp et al., 1998). Compared to non-users, MA users demonstrate cognitive impairment on recall tasks, ability to manipulate information, ability to ignore irrelevant information, and fluid intelligence (Halkitis, Parsons and Stirratt, 2001; Simon et al., 2000). Evidence suggests these effects can be long-term (Volkow et al., 2001a; 2001b). The drug is highly addictive, and abuse can result in aggressive behavior, paranoia, and potential neurological damage (Drug Enforcement Administration, 2000; National Institute on Drug Abuse, 2001). HIV infection and methamphetamine dependence are each associated with neuropsychological deficits, and these factors in combination are associated with an increased risk for developing HIV dementia (Rippeth et al., 2004). Many of these symptoms have the potential to become barriers for the client to engage fully in treatment. It has been the author's experience that those who are dependent on MA are less likely to recognize that their drug use is related to adverse life consequences until they are further into the dependence syndrome than for other drugs.

There are a variety of psychiatric symptoms that are commonly seen among methamphetamine users, with more severe symptoms occurring for those who use the drug with high intensity. Zweben et al. (2004) describes a clinical syndrome that includes mood disorders and suicidal behaviors as well as psychotic symptoms such as paranoia and hallucinations. While more extreme symptoms, such as acute psychosis tend to resolve shortly after cessation of methamphetamine, depressive symptoms tend to persist. Severe mood disturbance that last over a long period have the potential to affect a client's motivation for treatment. Depressed mood is a significant factor and may have a dramatic impact on motivation. Mood may improve relatively quickly, or it may take several months before mood returns to relatively normal levels (Newton et al., 2004).

Cravings associated with methamphetamine are reported to be stronger than other drugs, and result from dysphoria experienced once abstinence has been initiated (Rawson et al., 2002a). Cravings can be evoked through classical conditioning and occur when the client is exposed to internal or external cues. Strength of cravings is associated with the likelihood of relapse and those that continue to experience cravings well into abstinence have a higher likelihood of returning to methamphetamine (Littleton, 2000). Because the craving can be so intense during initial periods of abstinence, for those who are unable to go without using for even short periods of time, Rawson et al. (2002a) suggest that inpatient hospitalization is sometimes required for initial stages of detoxification and/or early abstinence.

Just as with others presenting for substance abuse treatment, MA users present with very strong ambivalence about quitting–often they desperately want to quit, but are unable to do so. Some may be ready to abstain from MA, while others may still want to moderate their use or are unsure of their desire or ability to stop. The Transtheoretical Model, which includes the "stages of change model," provides a way to conceptualize the extreme ambivalence associated with quitting methamphetamine. Clinicians should keep in mind that not everyone is ready to stop using MA when they seek help and that ambivalence is a normal phase in the change process.

EVIDENCE BASED TREATMENT STRATEGIES

Although MA and cocaine users may be very different in terms of demographic and drug use patterns, research suggests that response to outpatient treatment does not differ significantly (Rawson, 1998). Treatment strategies that have been empirically tested are based mostly on research conducted with stimulant disorders generally, but not MA disorders specifically. At this time, the most effective treatments for stimulant addiction are cognitive behavioral interventions (Cognitive Behavioral Therapy or CBT). Although there is little empirical support for 12 step recovery groups focusing on MA, many clinicians see crystal meth anonymous (CMA) as important in helping the client progress toward long-term drug-free recovery.

CBT incorporates a variety of strategies based on social learning principles and classical and operant conditioning. It may include identifying a number of factors that contribute to the initiation or continued use of MA. The assessment process used to identify these factors is commonly referred to as a "functional analysis," which helps the clinician and the client better understand in detail what function(s) MA serves for the client. One of the more important elements of CBT includes identifying antecedents of use, which means determining people, places and things that are likely to trigger use. Once risky situations that the client is likely to encounter are identified, CBT involves learning and reinforcing behavioral skills to avoid with cravings when possible and to cope with them once they arise if they are unavoidable. For most individuals who have substance use disorders, cognitive distortions are relatively common and CBT can be used to identify and challenge maladaptive cognitions. Additionally, CBT involves cognitive mediators of use, including having the client evaluate the positive and adverse consequences of use.

Motivational Interviewing (MI) is also increasingly being used as a tool to help those seeking treatment for substance use disorders and can be very helpful in managing the resistance, ambivalence, and lack of objective self-assessment that are common, particularly among those in the earlier stages of behavior change (Miller and Rollnick, 1991; DiClemente and Prochaska, 1998). While MI methods have been examined in multiple populations, and particularly among substance abusing populations (Bien, Miller and Tonigan, 1993; DiClemente, Bellino and Neavins, 1999; Dunn, Deroo and Rivara, 2001), they have not been tested as a stand-alone treatment for MA. However, MI has been used successfully to enhance adherence in outpatient cocaine treatment (Stotts, 2001) and has been used in combination with other treatment strategies (Shoptaw, 1997). MI can also be a helpful tool in the initial stages of treatment as an effective method of initiating treatment with clients who are unsure of goals.

One of the more effective treatments for stimulant use disorders is Community Reinforcement (CR) with adjunctive contingency management (CM). Combined CR/CM programs have been shown to be more effective than standard counseling strategies in both retaining clients significantly longer and documenting significantly longer periods of continuous stimulant abstinence (Amass, 1997; Higgins et al., 1993, 1994, 1995, 1997; Sisson and Azrin, 1989; Rawson et al., 2002b). The CR model incorporates a number of counseling and psychoeducational components, which may include couples therapy, vocational assistance, developing social support and cognitive behavioral skills training. As with many treatment strategies for MA use disorder, the CR model emphasizes the importance of treating alcohol use and other drug use disorders when present. Contingency management, which is often incorporated into CR, is a behavioral intervention that is designed to decrease MA use by providing reinforcement for clean urine toxicology results. It can be a very effective component of treatment for MA or other types of substance use disorders, because it sets concrete goals and can be used to recognize and emphasize behavioral changes.

For individuals who have been able to abstain from MA for a period of time, Relapse Prevention (Marlatt and Gordon, 1985) can help clients learn how to cope with substance craving, substance refusal and assertiveness skills; how seemingly irrelevant decisions can affect the probability of later substance use; general coping and problem solving skills; how to apply strategies to prevent a full-blown relapse should an episode of substance use occur. Relapse prevention has been shown to be useful with other substance use disorders and is superior to case management in reducing cocaine use (Carroll et al., 1994).

The Matrix Model (MM) is a treatment based on CBT principles that was developed specifically for stimulant abuse and dependence (Rawson et al., 2002b). The model integrates treatment elements from a number of specific strategies, including relapse prevention, motivational interviewing, psychoeducation, family therapy, and 12-Step program involvement. One unique aspect of the MM is that it has been adapted and tested with gay and bisexual men with stimulant use disorders. The goals of the Matrix Model include the following: stop drug use; teach clients issues critical to addiction and relapse; provide education for significant others affected by addiction and recovery; involve participants with self-help programs (CMA/AA); and reinforce negative urine toxicology and breathalyzer alcohol screens. The MM has been shown to reduce MA/cocaine use and has demonstrated to be effective in reducing HIV/STI related sexual risk behavior (Rawson et al., 1989, 1990, 1993; Huber et al., 1997; Shoptaw et al., 1994, 1997, 2005).

Regardless of the type of treatment that is delivered, a highly structured program is extremely important, particularly in the early stages of the treatment process. Rawson et al. (2002a) suggest a minimum of 3 visits per week for the first three months of treatment, but up to 5 visits per week is recommended. During months 3 through 6, 2 to 3 sessions per week are suggested. A combination of individual and group therapy can help to provide an individualized treatment program that also allows clients to understand that they share a common experience with others. The Center for Substance Abuse Treatment (Rawson, 1998) has published clinical recommendations for the treatment of methamphetamine called "CSAT Tip #33: Treatment of stimulant abuse" which provides a very good introduction regarding how to structure the treatment of stimulant dependence.

Methamphetamine, Sexual Compulsivity, and Other Drugs

For many individuals, MA use is inextricably tied to sexual behavior, regardless of sexual orientation. As mentioned above, however, among gay and bisexual men in urban areas there are many environments that specifically allow for both MA use and connecting with other users for sex. For those MSM entering recovery, it is extremely common to have engaged in a variety of MA fueled sexual compulsivity, which may include compulsive masturbation, compulsive sex with anonymous partners, pornography, Internet pornography and/or hook-ups as well as many other sexual outlets (Shoptaw and Frosch, 2000). Thus, of primary importance for clients entering treatment is to recognize that sexual thoughts and feelings can serve as triggers to returning to MA use. Because of the strong associations between sex and drugs that have developed for these individuals, temporary abstinence from sex may be helpful during initial treatment. Effective treatment programs should provide a safe environment for such clients to talk about these issues, either within the context of a group session or individual counseling. Additionally, clinicians should be aware that many who enter treatment may need to be tested for HIV and other STIs. Clinicians must be familiar with and comfortable with discussing risk behaviors and help clients set goals.

Most gay/bisexual men who use MA use it with other drugs (Halkitis, 2004). Use of other drugs can be a powerful trigger to return to MA and has to be addressed in treatment. Frequently, other drugs are used to manage the adverse effects of MA: benzodiazepines being used to go to sleep or taking Ecstasy (MDMA) to enhance MA's effect when going out to a club. It is not uncommon for those seeking treatment for MA to want to continue using other substances and to not see problems associated with their use. If possible, it is important to convey to the client that other drugs (including alcohol) can serve as triggers to return to MA. If this idea is met with resistance, it can sometimes be helpful to discuss immediate rather than long term goals for other drug use and, if possible, to have clients agree not to use for 90 days or some other agreed-upon period of time.

Methamphetamine and the Abstinence/Harm Reduction Debate

It is the author's experience that moderation is often a choice for those in earlier stages of change. However, few clinicians with experience treating MA dependence would suggest that it is easy or even possible to use the drug moderately. Clients who are MA dependent need to hear from professionals that moderation is unlikely to be successful and that abstinence is safer and easier. While the decision to abstain or to moderate is ultimately in the hands of the client, clinicians do have a responsibility to inform their clients about chances of success and failure of a given path. If clients are unwilling to stop altogether, it is important to reduce the harm associated with use when possible.

CONCLUSION

It is important that clinicians who refer their clients to methamphetamine treatment understand that the process can be very successful. It is even more important that they convey this to their clients. The current media attention has the potential to deter those who might be interested in treatment. The facts are that treatment success from MA has not been shown to be different than for other stimulants, such as cocaine, and that many people do recover if they are willing to commit to a structured treatment plan. It is very important that clinicians have a working knowledge of the contexts in which methamphetamine is used among gay and bisexual men and that they can participate in a frank dialogue with clients regarding the sexual behaviors and other factors that are associated with methamphetamine use.

REFERENCES

Amass, L. (1997), Financing voucher programs for pregnant substance abusers through community donations. In: *Problems of Drug Dependence 1996: Proceedings of the 58th Annual Scientific Meeting of the College on Problems of Drug Dependence*, ed. L.S. Harris (NIDA Research Monograph Series, Number 174. DHHS Pub. No. (ADM) 97-4236). Rockville, MD: National Institute on Drug Abuse, p. 60.

Benotsch, E.G., Kalichman, S.C. & Pinkerton, S.D. (2001), Sexual compulsivity in HIV positive men and women: Prevalence, predictors, and consequences of high risk behavior. *Sexual Addiction & Compulsivity*, 8(2):83-99.

Bien, T.H., Miller, W.R. & Tonigan, S.J. (1993), Brief interventions for alcohol problems: A review. *Addiction*, 88:315-336.

Carroll, K.M., Rounsaville, B.J., Gordon, L.T., Nich, C., Jatlow, P., Bisighini, R.M. & Gawin, F.H. (1994), Psychotherapy and pharmacotherapy for ambulatory cocaine abusers. *Archives General Psychiatry*, 51:177-187.

Colfax, G.N., Mansergh, G., Guzman, R., Vittinghoff, E., Marks, G., Rader, M. & Buchbinder, S. (2001), Drug use and sexual risk behavior among gay and bisexual men who attend circuit parties: A venue-based comparison. *J. Acquired Immune Deficiency Syndrome*, 28(4):373-9.

DiClemente, C.C. & Prochaska, J.O. (1998), Toward a comprehensive, theoretical model of change: Stages of change and addictive behaviors. In: *Treating Addictive Behaviors (2nd edition)*, eds. W.R. Miller & N. Heather. New York: Plenum Press, pp. 3-24.

DiClemente, C.C., Bellino, L.E. & Neavins, T.M. (1999), Motivation for change and alcoholism treatment. *Alcohol Research & Health*, 23(2):86-92.

Drug Enforcement Administration (DEA) (2000), *An Overview of Club Drugs*. Washington, DC: Drug Intelligence Brief, February.

Dunn, C., Deroo, L. & Rivara, F.P. (2001), The use of brief interventions adapted from motivational interviewing across behavioural domains: A systematic review. *Addiction*, 96:1725-1742.

Fernandez. (2004), NIDA Principal Investigator Meeting for drug use disorders among men who have sex with men. March 2004.

Halkitis, P.N., Parsons, J.T. & Stirratt, M. (2001), A double epidemic: Crystal methamphetamine use and its relation to HIV transmission among gay men. *J. Homosexuality*, 41(2), 17-35.

Higgins, S.T. & Budney, A.J. (1993), Treatment of cocaine dependence through the principles of behavior analysis and behavioral pharmacology. In: *Behavioral Treatments for Drug Abuse and Dependence*, eds. L.S. Onken, J.D. Blaine & J.J. Boren (NIDA Research Monograph Series, Number 137. NTIS Pub. No. 94-169570). Rockville, MD: National Institute on Drug Abuse, pp. 97-121.

Higgins, S.T. & Budney, A.J. (1997), From the initial clinic contact to aftercare: A brief review of effective strategies for retaining cocaine abusers in treatment. In: *Beyond the Therapeutic Alliance: Keeping the Drug-Dependent Individual in Treatment*, eds. L.S. Onken, J.D. Blaine & J.J. Boren (NIDA Research Monograph Series, Number 165. DHHS Pub. No. (ADM) 97-4142). Rockville, MD: National Institute on Drug Abuse, pp. 25-43.

Higgins, S.T., Budney, A.J., Bickel, W.K., Foerg, F.E. & Badger, G.J. (1994), Alcohol dependence and simultaneous cocaine and alcohol use in cocaine-dependent patients. *J. Addictive Diseases*, 13:177-189.

Higgins, S.T., Budney, A.J., Bickel, W.K., Foerg, F.E., Ogden, D. & Badger, G.J. (1995), Outpatient behavioral treatment for cocaine dependence: One-year outcome. *Experimental & Clinical Psychopharmacology*, 3:205-212.

Huber, A., Ling, W., Shoptaw, S., Gulati, V., Brethen, P. & Rawson, R. (1997), Integrating treatments for methamphetamine abuse: A psychosocial perspective. *J. Addictive Diseases*, 16(4):41-50.

Littleton, J. (2000), Can craving be modeled in animals? The relapse prevention perspective. *Addiction*, 95:S83-90.

Mansergh, G., Colfax, G.M., Marks, G., Rader, M., Guzman, R. & Buchbinder, S. (2001), The Circuit Party Men's Health Survey: Findings and implications for gay and bisexual men. *American J. Public Health*, 91(6):953-958.

Marlatt, G. & Gordon, J.R., eds. (1985), *Relapse Prevention: Maintenance Strategies in the Treatment of Addictive Behaviors*. New York: Guilford Press.

Miller, W.R. (1995), Increasing Motivation for change. In: *Handbook of Alcoholism Treatment Approaches: Effective Alternatives*, eds. R.K. Hester & W.R. Miller. Boston: Allyn and Bacon, pp. 89-104.

National Institute on Drug Abuse (NIDA) (2001), *Methamphetamine*. Bethesda, MD: U.S. Department of Health and Human Services. NIDA Infofax.

Newton, T.F., Kalechstein, A.D., Duran, S., Vansluis, N. & Ling, W. (2004), Methamphetamine abstinence syndrome: Preliminary findings. *American J. Addictions*, 13:248-255.

Rawson, R. (1998), *Treatment of Stimulant Abuse, CSAT Tip #33* (Chair, CSAT Consensus Panel). Rockville, MD: Department of Health and Human Services.

Rawson, R.A., Gonzales, R. & Brethen, P. (2002a), Treatment of methamphetamine use disorders: An update. *J. Substance Abuse Treatment*, 23(2):145-50.

Rawson, R.A., Huber, A., McCann, M., Shoptaw, S., Farabee, D., Reiber, C. & Ling, W. (2002b), A comparison of contingency management and cognitive-behavioral approaches during methadone maintenance treatment for cocaine dependence. *Archives General Psychiatry*, 59(9):817-824.

Rawson, R.A., Obert, J.L., McCann, M.J. & Castro, F.G (1991), Cocaine abuse treatment: A review of current strategies. *J. Substance Abuse*, 3(4):457-491.

Rawson, R.A., Obert, J.L., McCann, M.J. & Ling, W. (1993). Neurobehavioral treatment for cocaine dependency: A preliminary evaluation. In: *Cocaine Treatment: Research and Clinical Perspectives*, eds. F.M. Tims & C.G. Leukefeld (NIDA Research Monograph Series, Number 135. DHHS Pub. No. (ADM) 93-3639). Rockville, MD: National Institute on Drug Abuse, pp. 92-115.

Rawson, R.A., Obert, J.L., McCann, M.J., Smith, D.P. & Scheffy. (1990), Neurobehavioral treatment for cocaine dependency. *J. Psychoactive Drugs*, 22(2):159-171.

Rawson, R.A., Shoptaw, S.J., Obert, J.L., McCann, M.J., Hasson, A.L., Marinelli-Casey, P.J., Brethen, P.R. & Ling, W. (1995), An intensive outpatient approach for cocaine abuse treatment: The Matrix model. *J. Substance Abuse Treatment*, 12(2): 117-127.

Reback, C. (1997), *The Social Construction of a Gay Drug: Methamphetamine Use Among Gay and Bisexual Males in Los Angeles*. Los Angeles: City of Los Angeles, AIDS Coordinator.

Rippeth, J.D., Heaton, R.K., Carey, C.L., Marcotte, T.D, Moore, D.J., Gonzalez, R., Wolfson, T. & Grant, I. (2004), Methamphetamine dependence increases risk of neuropsychological impairment in HIV infected persons. *J. International Neuropsychological Society*, 10(1):1-14.

Semple, S.J., Patterson, T.L. & Grant, I. (2002), Motivations associated with methamphetamine use among HIV+ men who have sex with men. *J. Substance Abuse Treatment*, 22(3):149-56.

Shoptaw, S., Frosch, D., Rawson, R.A. & Ling, W. (1997), Cocaine abuse counseling as HIV protection. *AIDS Education & Prevention*, 9(6):511-520.

Shoptaw, S. & Frosch, D. (2000), Substance abuse treatment as HIV prevention for men who have sex with men. *AIDS & Behavior*, 4:193-203.

Shoptaw, S., Rawson, R.A., McCann, M.J. & Obert, J.L. (1994), The matrix model of outpatient stimulant abuse treatment: Evidence of efficacy. *J. Addictive Diseases*, 13(4):129-141.

Shoptaw, S., Reback, C.J., Peck, J.A., Yang X., Rotheram-Fuller E., Larkins S., Veniegas, R.C., Freese, T.E. & Hucks-Ortiz, C. (2005), Behavioral treatment approaches for methamphetamine dependence and HIV-related sexual risk behaviors among urban gay and bisexual men. *Drug & Alcohol Dependence*, 78(2):125-134.

Simon, S.L., Domier, C., Carnell, J., Brethen, P., Rawson, R. & Ling, W. (2000), Cognitive impairment in individuals currently using methamphetamine. *American J. Drug Addictions*, 9:222-231.

Stall, R., Paul, J.P., Greenwood, G., Pollack, L. M., Bein, E., Crosby, G.M., Mills, T.C., Binson, D., Coates, T.J. & Catania, J.A. (2001), Alcohol use, drug use and alcohol-related problems among men who have sex with men: The Urban Men's Health Study. *Addiction*, 96:1589-1601.

Stotts, A.L., Schmitz, J. M., Rhoades, H. M. & Grabowski, J. (2001), Motivational interviewing with cocaine-dependent patients: A pilot study. *J. Consulting & Clinical Psychology*, 69:858-862.

Tourangeau, R. & Smith, T.W. (1996), Asking sensitive questions: The impact of data collection mode, question format, and question context. *Public Opinion Quarterly*, 60(2):275-304.

Turner, C.F., Ku, L., Rogers, S.M., Lindberg, L.D. & Pleck, J.H. (1998), Adolescent sexual behavior, drug use, and violence: Increased reporting with computer survey technology. *Science*, 280:867-873.

Van Gorp, W., Altshuler, L., Theberge, D.C., Wilkins, J. & Dixon, W. (1998), Cognitive impairment in euthymic bipolar patients with and without prior alcohol dependence. *Archives General Psychiatry*, 55(1):41-46.

Volkow, N.D., Chang, L., Wang, G.J., Fowler, J.S., Franceschi, D., Sedler, M.J., Gatley, S.J., Hitzemann, R., Ding, Y.S., Wong, C. & Logan, J. (2001a), Higher cortical and lower subcortical metabolism in detoxified methamphetamine abusers. *American J. Psychiatry*, 158:383-389.

Volkow, N.D., Chang, L., Wang, G.J., Fowler, J.S., Leonido-Yee, M., Franceschi, D., Sedler, M.J., Gatley, S.J., Hitzemann, R., Ding, Y.S., Logan, J., Wong, C. & Miller, E.N. (2001b), Association of dopamine transporter reduction with psychomotor impairment in methamphetamine abusers. *American J. Psychiatry*, 158:377-383.

Zweben J.E., Cohen J.B., Christian D., Galloway, G.P., Salinardi, M., Parent, D. & Iguchi, M. (2004), Psychiatric symptoms in methamphetamine users. *American J. Addictions*, 13, 181-190.

Combining Motivational Interviewing and Cognitive-Behavioral Skills Training for the Treatment of Crystal Methamphetamine Abuse/Dependence

Donald A. Bux Jr., PhD
Thomas W. Irwin, PhD

SUMMARY. Methamphetamine addiction in men having sex with men (MSM) represents a particular challenge to the clinician. It requires attention both to the fundamental skills the client needs to acquire in order to attain abstinence, and to the client's level of motivation to change his behavior. What follows is a brief review of the state of the art of Motivational Interviewing (MI) and Cognitive-Behavioral Therapy (CBT) for addictions in general, and for crystal meth specifically. Much of the material presented here is not specific to treatment of crystal meth addiction in gay men; however, there are some aspects of treatment that are specific to treating crystal problems in MSM that are highlighted through-

Donald A. Bux Jr., is Research Associate, National Center on Addiction and Substance Abuse, Columbia University.

Thomas W. Irwin is Assistant Professor, Columbia University School of Medicine.

Address correspondence to: Donald A. Bux Jr., PhD, National Center on Addiction and Substance Abuse, Columbia University, 633 Third Avenue, 19th Floor, New York, NY 10017 (E-mail: dbux@casacolumbia.org).

[Haworth co-indexing entry note]: "Combining Motivational Interviewing and Cognitive-Behavioral Skills Training for the Treatment of Crystal Methamphetamine Abuse/Dependence." Bux, Donald A., Jr., and Thomas W. Irwin. Co-published simultaneously in *Journal of Gay & Lesbian Psychotherapy* (The Haworth Medical Press, an imprint of The Haworth Press, Inc.) Vol. 10, No. 3/4, 2006, pp. 143-152; and: *Crystal Meth and Men Who Have Sex with Men: What Mental Health Care Professionals Need to Know* (ed: Milton L. Wainberg, Andrew J. Kolodny, and Jack Drescher) The Haworth Medical Press, an imprint of The Haworth Press, Inc., 2006, pp. 143-152. Single or multiple copies of this article are available for a fee from The Haworth Document Delivery Service [1-800-HAWORTH, 9:00 a.m. - 5:00 p.m. (EST). E-mail address: docdelivery@haworthpress.com].

out this paper. This paper goes on to present the rationale and basic strategies encompassed by both motivation enhancement and skills-based treatment approaches. *[Article copies available for a fee from The Haworth Document Delivery Service: 1-800-HAWORTH. E-mail address: <docdelivery@haworthpress.com> Website: <http://www.HaworthPress.com> © 2006 by The Haworth Press, Inc. All rights reserved.]*

KEYWORDS. Addiction, cognitive-behavioral therapy, crystal methamphetamine, gay men, homosexuality, men having sex with men, motivation enhancement, motivation interviewing, skills-based treatment

What follows is a brief review of the state of the art of Motivational Interviewing (MI) and Cognitive-Behavioral Therapy (CBT) for addictions in general, and for crystal specifically. Much of the material presented here is not specific to treatment of crystal meth addiction in gay men; however, there are some aspects of treatment that are specific to treating crystal problems in men having sex with men (MSM) that are highlighted throughout this paper.

According to the cognitive behavioral model of addiction and recovery, there are three key factors that mediate recovery from substance abuse: motivation or readiness for change, self-efficacy-that is, the individual's estimation of the likelihood that he or she will succeed in changing should he or she decide to do so–and the development and successful implementation of skills for coping with the temptation to use. Consequently, treatment itself is likely to comprise two primary sets of strategies: motivation enhancement, and skills training.

MOTIVATIONAL INTERVIEWING

Key Points

Clinicians should be mindful of several key themes when implementing motivation enhancement techniques (Miller and Rollnick, 1991). First, it is taken as a given that clients entering substance abuse treatment are somewhat ambivalent about changing their behavior. That is, even though they might present with very compelling reasons for giving up substance use, they are likely to be harboring some equally compelling reasons for not doing so. This may be especially true for users of crystal meth, which can have both catastrophic negative consequences as well as intensely compelling positive effects. Thus the clinician implementing motivational techniques reacts to this ambivalence by validating both aspects of the client's experience, rather than attempting to negate, criticize or minimize the client's report of positive associations with crystal meth.

A second key theme of motivation enhancement approaches is that the client is viewed as both the one responsible for making decisions concerning change and as the agent of making change. What this means is that the treatment goal is not imposed on the client. A blanket requirement of abstinence as a goal is not consistent with motivational techniques. This is not to say that a non-abstinence goal is necessarily an appropriate or even achievable goal for most methamphetamine addicts; indeed in the authors' experience such a goal is highly unlikely. However, motivation enhancement is based on the presumption that clients who develop their own goals for treatment, and make their own decisions concerning how to accomplish those goals, will "own" the decision and the entire recovery process to a greater degree than clients who adopt a goal imposed by the clinician. Moreover, a failure to accomplish a non-abstinence goal that the client has selected can be framed by the clinician as a learning experience, and used as the basis of a re-evaluation of the treatment goal.

The third primary aspect of motivation enhancement is the avoidance of confrontation as a clinical strategy. Motivation enhancement, by striving to rely exclusively on non-confrontational interventions, aims to create a treatment context in which the client feels free to explore ambivalence concerning his behavior, and helps to reduce the defensiveness that inevitably results when that ambivalence is directly challenged. This runs contrary to the impulse to confront denial, especially in severely dependent users, where the problems associated with use are often all too clear to the clinician. However, it is vital to the clinical process in motivation enhancement therapy that the client feel free to voice his ambivalence, including his concerns and fears about the costs he perceives of reducing or eliminating use. For example, whereas in more traditional settings a client's expression of uncertainty regarding the need for abstinence might elicit a comment on the client's denial, in motivation enhancement the clinician responds by validating that experience with an empathic, reflective statement (e.g., "So you're really not even convinced that there's a problem here."). This strategy is intended to give the client "space" to articulate all aspects of his experience, rather than risk increasing his defensiveness and resistance as a reaction to the clinician's criticism.

Information Gathering

The first step in motivation enhancement is to gather a detailed history of the client's substance use, his current pattern of use, and critical points in the history such as marked changes in the pattern, frequency, route of administration, or type of substances used. The therapist uses carefully crafted questions to guide the discussion without giving the impression of having an "agenda" (i.e., proving that the client has a problem). The goal is to help the client chart his path of use, and in particular to note points at which use increased, or at which his behavior crossed a "line in the sand"; that is, occasions on which he did things that he might previously have believed he would never do (e.g., using during the week, or injecting versus smoking or snorting). Information about consequences of use is also sought here, but such questions should be balanced with questions about the positive aspects of use, in order to maintain as neutral a stance as possible and foster open communication in the session. Again, the goal is to create an environment in which the client feels comfortable to divulge information about consequences rather than being pressed to do so; if this atmosphere is not provided, the client may fear being "cornered" and may thus withhold or minimize information about the problems he is experiencing. Thus this strategy is intended to help minimize defensiveness and denial, by allowing the client to proceed at his own pace.

It is also important to highlight periods during which the client was abstinent from use for any length of time, to help lay the foundation for building self-efficacy; that is, the client's internal sense that he is capable of accomplishing and sustaining change. Questions about the circumstances of such periods, strategies used to attain abstinence, and circumstances surrounding the return to use can all be useful in this context.

Key Principles

Four overarching principles govern the therapist's behavior in motivation enhancement. The first, alluded to above, is expression of empathy. The therapist should always convey a sympathetic understanding of the client's perspective, regardless of what that perspective is. This does not necessarily mean the provider needs to *approve of* or *agree with* that perspective, but it is essential that the therapist always demonstrate that he or she accepts what the client has to say as a valid point of view.

The second principle is the development of discrepancy. This refers to the process by which the client comes to evaluate fully his pattern of behavior and its consequences, both good and bad, and to consider these in the context of his self-image and larger life goals. This discrepancy between current behavior and the "ideal self" can be the driving force behind the decision to change. It is worth noting that the development of discrepancy is often at odds with a basic instinct of therapists: to make clients feel more comfortable. When discrepancy is high, clients feel uncomfortable and in distress, but unlike the use of confrontational techniques (where the client has an obvious target to blame for his discomfort, and thus tends to react with defensiveness), motivational techniques attempt to ensure that the source of the client's discrepancy is wholly internal.

The third principle of motivation enhancement is "rolling with resistance" and avoiding argumentation. As already noted, direct confrontation or argumentation with a client often provokes a defensive or resistant reaction. By providing an empathic response to resistance (e.g., "It sounds like you're really not sure you need to make any changes at all") instead of a confrontational one ("You really seem to be minimizing the problems you're having"), the therapist reduces the possibility of defensive or resistant responses, and instead invites the client either to elaborate on his or her doubts, or to respond with a statement expressing the other side of the ambivalence ("Well, I know there's a problem; I'm just not sure how much of a change I need to make").

The fourth key principle of motivation enhancement is supporting self-efficacy. A primary source of uncertainty about change in substance abuse is often the client's doubts about success. The therapist's goal in motivation enhancement is to help the client explore these doubts and challenge them (see below).

Key Strategies

Three key strategies are useful in accomplishing the goals described above. The first of these is a set of basic clinical skills collectively referred to by the acronym, "OARS," which refers to *Open questions, Affirmations, Reflective listening*, and *Summary statements*.

Open questions solicit information about the client's perspective on his or her substance use, without communicating any judgments or preconceptions on the part of the therapist. These questions are not answerable with a one-word, yes-or-no response; they require thought and reflection on the part of the client. Genuine *affirmations* reinforce the client's strengths and convey the therapist's belief that the client has the capacity for change. They convey the therapist's enthusiasm for and faith in the client's intrinsic capabilities and provide needed encouragement in the change process. *Reflective listening* conveys the therapist's understanding of the client, and helps draw out more information in a non-threatening manner. It can also guide the discussion further if used to amplify a particular aspect of what the client is saying. *Summary statements* are used by the therapist to tie together disparate pieces of information and contradictory statements from the client, in order to help the client evaluate his or her ambivalence and help build discrepancy.

The second key strategy in motivation enhancement is the elicitation of "change talk" and "commitment talk." The therapist aims to elicit "DARN-C" statements from the client, that indicate the client's *Desire* to, *Ability* to, *Reasons* for, *Need* for, and *Commitment* to change. This in turn is accomplished through a variety of strategies; for example, statements that summarize both sides of the client's ambivalence, followed by questions that press the client to resolve the apparent contradiction.

The third key strategy is the deflection of resistance, and includes a number of specific interventions. In response to a statement from a client indicative of resistance to change (for example, the client states, "The thing is, I'm just not so far gone like some of the guys I see who have real problems"), the therapist might respond with a *simple reflection*, which refers to answering the statement with a reflection indicating acceptance of his viewpoint, which is intended to validate the client's perspective and give him "space" to consider the other, possibly more threatening side of his ambivalence (e.g., "So you're not sure how bad a problem this is right now"). An alternative can be an *amplified reflection*, or taking a mildly resistant statement from a client and magnifying it, thereby encouraging the client to back away from the resistance and argue in favor of change (e.g., "So what you're basically saying is that everything's under control and there's nothing at all to be concerned about here"). A more sophisticated strategy is the *double-sided reflection*, which involves reflecting what the client has just said, then linking it to other material the client has previously provided that is supportive of change, in a "on the one hand . . . on the other hand . . ." manner (e.g., "So while you're saying here that the crystal certainly could be a bigger problem than it is, you're still concerned that you're using more, you've missed work twice, and you've had unsafe sex several times in the past couple of months").

COGNITIVE-BEHAVIORAL TREATMENT: SKILLS TRAINING

Principles

The key principle underlying skills training approaches is that recovery is a learning process. Clients achieve recovery by learning specific skills and strategies for managing addiction. These include challenging the client's self-defeating beliefs about his incapacity for avoiding or controlling use, coping skills for dealing with temptations to use, and challenging the client's expectations concerning the outcomes of substance use and abstinence (Marlatt and Gordon, 1985).

Enhancing Self-Efficacy

A key factor underlying low self-efficacy for abstinence is the client's often distorted perception concerning what abstinence will entail. It is therefore important to identify and challenge such distortions. Abstinence often seems an unimaginable, hypothetical state, one far removed from life as the client currently knows it. Helping the client to envision in detail a future without substance use, and to recall what his life was like before initiating substance use (if a sufficient adult life history without substance use is present), helps to de-mystify abstinence and make it seem more realistic.

Another strategy for addressing the perception of abstinence as an unimaginably large change from the present pattern of behavior is to help the client consider what changes are more immediately possible and attainable, rather than single-mindedly focusing on abstinence. Clients feel they are more able to accomplish the goal if it is broken down into smaller, more manageable steps. For example, a client who believes he is not yet capable of abstaining could be encouraged to start attending meetings of Crystal Meth Anonymous (if available), which could provide the foundation for a recovery-oriented social network that may facilitate abstinence down the road.

Clients often underestimate their own capacity for change, based on their prior and ultimately unsuccessful attempts to abstain from or moderate substance use. A detailed examination of such prior attempts is useful in helping clients to see them in less black-and-white, failure-not-success terms. Specifically, reviewing the circumstances under which the client achieved abstinence, the process behind the decision to abstain, the factors present in the client's life at the time that made the period of abstinence (however brief) possible, and the specific strategies the client used to facilitate abstinence will help him recognize the skills and strengths he may already have at his or her disposal for the next undertaking. This examination may also be used to help reframe prior relapses not as failures, but as learning experiences. Instead of focusing on "falling off the wagon," the client can be encouraged to consider "what went wrong," as a means of developing a better plan for the next attempt.

Addressing Expectancies

Expectancies for substance use are a powerful factor that can undermine treatment; their salience varies considerably depending on the circumstances in which the client finds himself. Although the client who is motivated to change may unequivocally articulate numerous negative outcomes of substance use, at times of high temptation to use, the latter may diminish in importance relative to positive expectancies of use. Clients therefore should be encouraged to identify all negative and positive outcomes associated with use. These can then be examined in detail, and their differences discussed. For example, it can be pointed out that positive outcomes of use are typically short-term and very salient during times of temptation (enhanced sex, escape from immediate stress, etc.), while negative outcomes are long-term and relatively remote in the individual's consciousness in high-risk situations. The client can then be encouraged to develop strategies for challenging positive expectancies of use when they come into consciousness.

Negative expectancies concerning abstinence are often overlooked in substance abuse treatment, but they are important to address because they often go unarticulated by the client if not specifically elicited. Nevertheless, clients often perceive substantial costs to giving up crystal meth. For some gay men in large urban centers, particularly, those for whom crystal is a significant aspect of their gay night life, the drug may be seen as a central part of the client's gay identity (Reback, 1997). To such a gay man, a substantial segment of gay life may appear inaccessible to him if crystal is given up. Similarly, the link between sex and crystal is very strong, and for the majority of gay men who use crystal to enhance sexual encounters ("party and play"), the idea of sex while sober is felt to be boring at best, and inconceivable at worst (Reback, 1997). Sex itself becomes a very powerful trigger for use, and often the biggest hurdle for gay men recovering from crystal addiction is learning new sexual scripts that do not include the drug, and for the gay man in early recovery giving up crystal may quite literally mean giving up his usual way of having sex.

Avoiding High-Risk Situations

The single most important skill the client acquires in cognitive-behavior therapy is how to cope with urges to use. Here, a multi-level approach is used to maximize successful coping. The first step involves identifying what situations are high-risk for the client, usually meaning those situations in which he has most typically used in the past ("people, places and things"). The client is encouraged to consider both internal cues (mood states, enabling thoughts–"just one bump won't hurt"–etc.) and external cues (certain friends, sexual situations, nightclubs, etc.). Next the client is encouraged to identify which situations he is able and willing to avoid outright (certain friends, nightclubs, Internet sex sites), and to develop a behavioral plan that will enable him to do so (e.g., cut off or reduce contact with drug using friends, adopting alternative leisure activities).

Coping with Urges

For those situations that the client is either unable (feeling depressed) or unwilling (sex, certain friends) to completely avoid, the client is encouraged to develop strategies for minimizing and coping with the urges that do arise. This includes teaching such skills as drug refusal and "urge surfing" (a strategy derived from Zen practices involving the visualization of an urge, that redirects the client's mental energy from the need to act on the urge to the simple observation of the urge). Other strategies include scheduling alternate activities that are incompatible with use (e.g., a visit to one's parents, seeing friends who use only in contexts where use is not practical), coping skills for dealing with depression and other negative affect, and specific skills for moderation management when the client does not endorse an abstinence goal. The client might explicitly seek sex partners who don't "party and play," or request in advance that the partner not use in his presence. Looking for sex partners on the Internet might be a context with a particularly high risk for use, and the client might be encouraged to find alternatives to this practice. As noted above, non-abstinence goals are not considered realistic for most dependent users of crystal; while it is appropriate for the therapist to convey this opinion, it is also important that the client remain engaged in treatment if he does not endorse this goal. An eventual failure in a moderation goal may then be used as information for the client concerning what his next step should be (i.e., consideration of an abstinence goal).

Coping with 'Slips'

The client needs to be prepared for setbacks. Thus, while the ultimate goal of treatment may be abstinence or substantial moderation, it is important that the client not give up if this goal proves difficult to achieve. Clients benefit from making a distinction between a "lapse" and a "relapse"; that is, between a single slip-up and a complete abandonment of efforts at recovery. Thus, they do not as easily fall into the trap of the "abstinence violation effect," which can lead the client to regard a slip as a failure, and in turn to abandon all efforts to recover. Clients should be encouraged to develop a coping plan for dealing with slips that includes an immediate renewal of commitment to the original treatment goal, and a review of the slip that allows it to become a learning experience.

REFERENCES/SUGGESTED READING

Marlatt, G.A. & Gordon, J.R. (1985), *Relapse Prevention.* New York: Guilford.

Miller, W.R. & Rollnick, S. (1991), *Motivational Interviewing: Preparing People to Change Addictive Behavior.* New York: Guilford.

Reback, C.J. (1997), *The social construction of a gay drug: Methamphetamine use among gay and bisexual men in Los Angeles.* Los Angeles: City of Los Angeles, AIDS Coordinator's Office.

Understanding and Treating the Crystal Methamphetamine Emerging Health Crisis: Using Community-Based Resources at the Lesbian, Gay, Bisexual and Transgender Community Center

Jean Malpas, MA, LMHC
Barbara E. Warren, PsyD, CASAC, CPP

SUMMARY. Recent research on crystal methamphetamine use among gay, bisexual and men who have sex with men (MSM) in the greater New York City metropolitan area indicates that crystal meth use is rising in this population and that it is correlated to increased risk for HIV, addiction, medical and mental disorders. Prevention and treatment of crystal meth related problems that are sensitive to the needs of MSM populations must be further developed to address this emerging crisis. Gay-identified community-based programs provide a viable resource

Jean Malpas was a counselor at the Lesbian, Gay, Bisexual and Transgender Community Center CARE (Counseling, Advocacy Recovery and Education) and is in private practice.

Barbara E. Warren is the Director for Organizational Development, Planning & Research at the Lesbian, Gay, Bisexual and Transgender Community Center.

Address correspondence to: Barbara E. Warren, the Center, 208 West 13th Street, New York City, NY 10011 (E-mail: BarbaraW@gaycenter.org).

[Haworth co-indexing entry note]: "Understanding and Treating the Crystal Methamphetamine Emerging Health Crisis: Using Community-Based Resources at the Lesbian, Gay, Bisexual and Transgender Community Center." Malpas, Jean, and Barbara E. Warren. Co-published simultaneously in *Journal of Gay & Lesbian Psychotherapy* (The Haworth Medical Press, an imprint of The Haworth Press, Inc.) Vol. 10, No. 3/4, 2006, pp. 153-157; and: *Crystal Meth and Men Who Have Sex with Men: What Mental Health Care Professionals Need to Know* (ed: Milton L. Wainberg, Andrew J. Kolodny, and Jack Drescher) The Haworth Medical Press, an imprint of The Haworth Press, Inc., 2006, pp. 153-157. Single or multiple copies of this article are available for a fee from The Haworth Document Delivery Service [1-800-HAWORTH, 9:00 a.m. - 5:00 p.m. (EST). E-mail address: docdelivery@haworthpress.com].

Available online at http://jglp.haworthpress.com
doi:10.1300/J236v10n03_14

within which to develop and deliver such services but will need more resources and funding to meet the growing demand. *[Article copies available for a fee from The Haworth Document Delivery Service: 1-800-HAWORTH. E-mail address: <docdelivery@haworthpress.com> Website: <http://www.HaworthPress.com>*
© 2006 by The Haworth Press, Inc. All rights reserved.]

KEYWORDS. AIDS, bisexual men, community based organization, crystal meth, gay men, harm reduction, HIV, homosexuality, men having sex with men (MSM), methamphetamine, substance abuse, transtheoretical model

During the early 1990s, research studies determined that crystal methamphetamine use was largely a regional phenomenon confined to the western portion of the United States. These earlier studies documented methamphetamine prevalence rates that ranged between 5% and 25% of the gay and bisexual men surveyed (Reback and Ditman, 1997).

More recently, Perry Halkitis, PhD's *Project TINA* and *Project BUMPS* studies at the Center for HIV/AIDS Education, Studies and Training (CHEST) in New York City have found that among New York City gay or bisexual male self-identified crystal methamphetamine users (n = 208), 62% of the participants indicated significant and frequent use of crystal methamphetamine (Halkitis and Parsons, 2002a). A substantial proportion of the men reported poly-drug use combining methamphetamine with alcohol (45%), with ecstasy [MDMA] (39%), with ketamine (32%), with Viagra [sildenafil] (29%), with inhalant nitrates (28%), and with cocaine (25%). In both studies, participants crossed lines of race/ethnicity, age, income, and HIV status. Ages of the participants ranged from 20 to 55; 45% of the sample were men of color; and half of the participants reported being HIV positive.

In the face of studies and statistics like these, the Lesbian, Gay, Bisexual and Transgender Center (the Center) is working with Gay Men's Health Crisis and Harlem United to address this growing problem. Specifically, our New York City LGBT Community Center's Center CARE (Counseling, Advocacy Recovery and Education) program has attempted to address the increased demand for assistance with crystal methamphetamine and other club/party drugs among both adolescent and adult gay and bisexual men. During 2003, Center CARE has treated over 100 men presenting with primary substance abuse or dependence on crystal methamphetamine; nearly double the number in 2002. Currently, 61 clients are actively receiving individual and group counseling at our Center.

Of these 61 clients, only one is female, 7 self-identify as Latino, 3 as African American and the rest as White.

To date, all Center CARE clients report as their preferred self-administration method either smoking or snorting; none have reported intravenous injection or booty-bumpers (anal insertion). Anecdotal evidence and data from the Drug Enforcement Administration points to an increase number of men using crystal via injection. Our clients' HIV status is evenly split between those who are negative and positive. As described in other research studies (Gorman, 1996; Gorman et al., 1996; Lewis and Ross, 1995), the Center's clients also present with several mental health disorders and other problems associated with crystal methamphetamine. These problems include HIV/AIDS-related issues, social phobias, anxiety, depression, bipolar disorder, attention deficit disorders, sexual compulsivity, social isolation, and a host of severe physical effects of the drug itself.

Specialized treatment centers for crystal methamphetamine are hard to find. Yet, standard substance abuse treatment is not effective for the treatment of crystal methamphetamine abuse or dependence (Rawson, 2004). In order to effectively treat clients who present at the Center, comprehensive psychosocial assessments and screening for co-presenting mental health concerns are conducted. The Center offers individual and group counseling–primarily short-term (10-12 weeks), guided by the transtheoretical model of behavioral change. This model delineates the cognitive processes involved as individuals move through stages of (1) awareness of the need to change; (2) considering the pros and cons of changing; (3) making a decision to attempt to change; (4) preparing to make a change; and (5) then acting upon and sustaining the change (Prochaska, 1992). In accordance with this model, participants are engaged using specific strategies to manage barriers, increase motivation and define skills to acquire the healthier behavior. The Center groups are structured to engage clients at their stage of readiness and guide them through this thinking process. In addition, Center CARE runs an open drop-in support group–*Come As You Are*–for men in contemplation and preparation; that is, those who have concerns about their drug use, but who are not quite ready to begin making changes. There is also a closed 12-week group, *Sex, Drugs and Recovery*, for men in the action and maintenance stages who need to build skills and support for recovery. Unfortunately, the Center currently has a two-week waiting list for an initial interview due to insufficient staff capacity to meet the growing demand.

The Center continues to do street outreach through the distribution of literature about the Center services in bars and clubs. In addition to distributing educational information in the monthly *Center Happenings*, ads are run in gay newspapers and posters are displayed in the Chelsea and Greenwich Village neighborhoods of Manhattan. The Center Website receives 60,000 visitors per month. In collaboration with CHEST, there is a Crystal Meth web page with information about crystal use and community resources. This web page also offers a specially designed self-administered educational, data collection and needs assessment survey. The survey was on-line as of February 2004 and the unduplicated number of visitors averages 700 per month. Over 300 completed surveys have been received and the first analysis of the data will be run at the end of 2005.

Given the high correlation between crystal methamphetamine use and unprotected sex (Halkitis and Parsons, 2002b), the necessity to intervene effectively around crystal methamphetamine is critical to preventing HIV transmission. In collaboration with other local organizations, we have developed community level interventions to increase community awareness; provide accurate information about risks; offer community resources and referrals; and build community support for recovery. These have included open forums: An Evening with Crystal, Drugs Are Us, and Sex in the City. They are co-hosted by the Center, Gay Men's Health Crisis (GMHC,) Dance Safe, Harm Reduction Coalition, HX magazine and CHEST and average 100 participants per forum,. Most recently, we have worked with Callen-Lorde Community Health Center and the HIV Forum providing outreach and space for several community forums focusing on HIV prevention and crystal methamphetamine use in our communities.

To continue to effectively address the growing crystal methamphetamine and other club/party drug crisis among gay and bisexual men–and among all young people in NYC–increased local capacity to respond both with prevention and intervention services is needed. A critical need is to recruit trained professionals at the community-based organization level, as well as to train current staff to offer a continuum of services with specific interventions for crystal methamphetamine and other club/party drug. It is important to offer specialized services at the community-based level and citywide in order to reach young adult and adult MSM who may not be willing to access traditional treatment settings that are not low threshold, or may not be sensitive to the issues these men face in partnering with other men.

Outreach must be tailored to specifically target populations of gay/bi men of color and men on the "down-low" (MSM who do not identify as gay or bisexual) using crystal. Toward this end, the Center has partnered with Harlem United Community AIDS Center to create education messages that are targeted to MSM of color as a prevention and early intervention initiative.

What is still needed is an increased capacity to collect data, to evaluate interventions for efficacy and to refine them accordingly, to conduct outreach and education campaigns citywide, and to train the mainstream substance abuse treatment programs and their staff about the specific interventions that are effective with crystal methamphetamine and other club/party drugs for the LGBT community.

REFERENCES

Gorman, M.E., Gunderson, R., Marlatt, A. & Donovan, D. (1996), *HIV Risk among Gay and Bisexual Methamphetamine Injectors in Seattle, Washington.* Presented at the International Conference on AIDS (ICA Abstracts, Pub.C., p. 1257).

Gorman, M. (1996), Speed use and HIV transmission. *Focus,* 11(7):4-8.

Halkitis, P.N. & Parsons, J.T. (2002a), *Methamphetamine Use among Gay and Bisexual Men in New York City.* Paper presented at the 4th Annual Harm reduction Conference, Seattle, WA, December.

Halkitis, P.N. & Parsons, J.T. (2002b), Recreational drug use and HIV risk sexual behavior among men frequenting urban gay venues. *J. Gay & Lesbian Social Services,* 14(4):19-39.

Halkitis, P.N., Parsons, J.T. & Stirratt, M. (2001), A double epidemic: Crystal methamphetamine use and its relation to HIV prevention among gay men. *J. Homosexuality, 41*(2):17-35.

Halkitis, P.N., Parsons, J.T. & Wilton, L. (2002), *Characteristics of Gay and Bisexual Methamphetamine Users and Contexts of Use in New York City.* Unpublished Manuscript.

Lewis, L.A. & Ross, M.W. (1995), The gay dance party culture in Sydney: A qualitative analysis. *J. Homosexuality,* 29(1):41-70.

Lewis, L.A. & Ross, M.W. (1995), *A Select Body: The Gay Dance Party Subculture and the HIV/AIDS Pandemic.* New York: Cassell Publications.

Prochaska, J.O., DiClemente, C.C. & Norcross, J.C. (1992), In search of how people change: Applications to addictive behaviors. *American Psychologist,* 47(9): 1102-1114.

Rawson, R.A., Marinelli-Casey, P., Anglin, M.D., Dickow, A., Frazier,Y., Gallagher, C., Galloway, G.P., Herrell, J., Huber, A., McCann, M.J., Obert, J., Pennell, S., Reiber, C., Vandersloot, D. & Zweben, J. (2004), A multi-site comparison of psychosocial approaches for the treatment of methamphetamine dependence. *Addiction,* 99:708-717.

Reback, C. & Ditman, D. (1997), *The Social Construction of a Gay Drug: Methamphetamine Use Among Gay and Bisexual Males in Los Angeles. Executive Summary.* City of Los Angeles, AIDS Coordinator. Los Angeles.

Harm Reduction, Crystal Methamphetamine, and Gay Men

L. Donald McVinney, MSSW, MPhil

SUMMARY. This article describes changing definitions and models of harm reduction along with their practice applications. This article then provides an overview of harm reduction strategies for methamphetamine-using gay men and will conclude with suggestions for psychotherapists and clinicians who are, or who will be, working with this population. *[Article copies available for a fee from The Haworth Document Delivery Service: 1-800-HAWORTH. E-mail address: <docdelivery@haworthpress.com> Website: <http://www.HaworthPress.com> © 2006 by The Haworth Press, Inc. All rights reserved.]*

KEYWORDS. AIDS, bisexual men, crystal meth, gay men, harm reduction, HIV, homosexuality, men having sex with men (MSM), methamphetamine substance abuse

Harm reduction is a contemporary perspective, or framework, for understanding drug use and drug users that can guide clinicians through a

L. Donald McVinney is National Director of Education and Training, Harm Reduction Coalition; and Adjunct Lecturer, Columbia University School of Social Work.

Address correspondence to: L. Donald McVinney, Harm Reduction Coalition, 22 West 27th Street, 5th Floor, New York, NY 10001 (E-mail: mcvinney@harmreduction.org; ldm3@columbia.edu).

[Haworth co-indexing entry note]: "Harm Reduction, Crystal Methamphetamine, and Gay Men." McVinney, L. Donald. Co-published simultaneously in *Journal of Gay & Lesbian Psychotherapy* (The Haworth Medical Press, an imprint of The Haworth Press, Inc.) Vol. 10, No. 3/4, 2006, pp. 159-169; and: *Crystal Meth and Men Who Have Sex with Men: What Mental Health Care Professionals Need to Know* (ed: Milton L. Wainberg, Andrew J. Kolodny, and Jack Drescher) The Haworth Medical Press, an imprint of The Haworth Press, Inc., 2006, pp. 159-169. Single or multiple copies of this article are available for a fee from The Haworth Document Delivery Service [1-800-HAWORTH, 9:00 a.m. - 5:00 p.m. (EST). E-mail address: docdelivery@haworthpress.com].

Available online at http://jglp.haworthpress.com
© 2006 by The Haworth Press, Inc. All rights reserved.
doi:10.1300/J236v10n03_15

broad range of available interventions. Because harm reduction is a perspective, or a way of viewing the impact of drug use on a person's psychosocial functioning, it is not bound to any one therapeutic theory of action and allows for various theoretical strategies to inform interventions (Tatarsky, 2002). Interventions that are guided by a harm reduction perspective can meet the needs of diverse clients who use an array of psychoactive substances. Gay men who use crystal meth, often in combination with other so-called "party drugs," may benefit from harm reduction strategies (http://www.tweaker.org; http://www.crystalneon.org; Kingston and Conrad, 2004).

A harm reduction perspective allows clinicians and drug users together to establish goals and objectives to reduce drug-related harm that is based on the notion of a client's right to self-determination. Harm reduction has emerged over the last fifteen years in the United States as the new paradigm for intervening with substance users. Harm reduction offers an alternative approach to what has been called "the moral model" (zero tolerance), the punitive criminal justice model (the war on drugs and incarceration), and the biomedical (disease) model that have dominated drug policy and drug treatment for the last half century in the United States (Des Jarlais, 1995).

HARM REDUCTION TERMINOLOGY

Various terms have been used to define the concept of harm reduction. For purposes of this article, the terms *harm minimization, risk reduction* and *harm elimination* are all subsumed within the concept of harm reduction (Roberts and Marlatt, 1999).

The definition of harm reduction has changed over time to meet the contemporary challenges of public policy and service delivery. Initially, harm reduction was defined within the context of a sub-population of drug users, those who injected; even today, many clinicians and policy makers continue to associate harm reduction exclusively with this population. More contemporaneous definitions reflect the broader scope of harm reduction and its application in diverse settings and communities. In the United States, the Harm Reduction Coalition (2005), the first national organization formed to address drug-related harm through education has developed the following working definition. According to the Coalition's website:

Harm reduction is an approach that aims to reduce the negative consequences of drug use through utilizing a full spectrum of strategies from safer drug use, to moderation, to abstinence. Oriented toward working with the whole person, harm reduction programs and policies create environments and develop strategies for change that are practical, humane and effective. These programs meet consumers "where they are at" to help them become more conscious of the harm in their lives and identify options for reducing those harms. The goal of these interventions and policies is to help people and communities maximize their health and potential while simultaneously reducing harm. While harm reduction is most commonly thought of as an approach to reducing drug-related harm, its philosophy and practice have applications for all professions and communities. (http://www.harmreduction.org)

Ongoing debates over the meaning of harm reduction and its practical applications are often framed as "abstinence versus harm reduction" when, in fact, abstinence is an excellent form of harm reduction (Zelvin and Davis, 2001). However, the goal of intervention may not necessarily be the cessation of drug use, particularly if that is not a goal of the client. In this model, goals are mutually agreed upon by clients and clinicians together and should be attainable. Harm reduction is a form of health promotion, since in reducing drug-related harm, or harmful drug-related behaviors, one is simultaneously promoting the health and well being of drug users. Harm reduction has been advocated across disciplines, in social work, nursing, and psychology (Bradley-Springer, 1996; Brocato and Wagner, 2003; Housenbold Seiger, 2003; MacCoun, 1998; Van Wormer and Davis, 2003).

CRYSTAL METH: THE SCOPE OF THE PROBLEM

A harm reduction perspective is being used quite effectively with crystal methamphetamine users. "Crystal" or "tina," as the drug is popularly known among gay men, poses challenges that are applicable to drug use across all categories. However, unique challenges are posed by this drug's pharmacology, the mindset or expectancy of crystal using gay men (who are referred to, not necessarily pejoratively, but often affectionately as "tweakers" and "crystal fairies") and the gay venues or settings in which it is used. Some of these challenges are presented below.

Studies have found a rise in crystal use across the U.S. over the last several years based upon (1) the number of people seeking treatment for crystal; (2) the number of people presenting to emergency departments; (3) the number of crystal methamphetamine arrests; and (4) methamphetamine lab seizures.

Crystal use among gay and bisexual men is an emerging social problem (Rebak, 1997). A review of the literature reveals an alarming rise of crystal use among gay men nationally (Halkitis, Parsons and Wilton, 2003; Reback, Larkins and Shoptaw, 2004; Semple, Patterson and Grant, 2003; Urbina and Jones, 2004). Gay-specific environments and subcultures are now often linked with crystal use; these include circuit parties, dance clubs, sex clubs/bathhouses, and chat rooms/internet hookups devoted to "PNP" ("Party and Play"), an identifier for sex-seeking crystal users (Owen, 2004). Based upon this author's experience, gay men report that there is not only much less stigma associated with crystal use, which used to have an association with rural poor whites, but that it has become the "chi-chi" drug at parties, openly used with a cachet that powdered cocaine used to have in the 1970s and 1980s. According to one recent study, anecdotal evidence from community-based organizations serving gay and bisexual men in New York City and in private practice (Guss, 2000) supports this report of increased methamphetamine use (Halkitis, Parsons and Wilton, 2003, p. 426). The same authors cited several studies that permitted them to conclude . . . "this investigation corroborates with both recent anecdotal and documented evidence suggesting that methamphetamine is emerging as a popular substance in New York City's gay community" (pp. 423-424).

In order for interventions to be effective, clinicians need to assess the mindset of the user and inquire about some of the reasons why a person is using crystal. The perceived beneficial or desired effects from crystal that are cited by gay men in this author's experience and in numerous studies (Freese, Miotto and Reback, 2002; Guss, 2000; Halkitis, Parsons and Wilton, 2003; Reback, Larkins and Shoptaw, 2004; Semple, Patterson and Grant, 2002; 2003; Shernoff, 2005) include:

- Provides energy and increases alertness
- Lessens desire and ability to sleep
- Increases stamina and enhances endurance (appeals to body builders)
- Reduces appetite and burns fat
- Induces sense of self-confidence and increases productivity
- Increases sexual desire and arousal

- Focuses thinking and increases concentration
- Distorts perceptions of time
- A form of escape from "hassles of daily living"
- Enhances and/or prolongs intensity and frequency of sexual encounters
- Keeps one awake for weekend-long parties
- Helps one escape from unpleasant emotions, which has been linked to avoidance of dealing with one's HIV status (Halkitis, Parsons and Wilton, 2003).

Harm reduction strategies may focus on the drug's powerful pharmacological effects on the user as a way to raise obvious discrepancies between the drug's perceived benefits and its risks. The adverse side effects of crystal include increased heart rate and blood pressure, induced shallow breathing, sweating, enlarged pupils, dry mouth, pounding headaches, and because of the increase in motor activity, risks of dehydration and malnourishment from not eating. Harm reduction strategies may encourage clients to "chill out" and give one's body a rest, to drink fluids and take time to eat and sleep (Gay Men's Health Crisis, 2004; http://www.tweaker.org; http://www.crystal neon.org).

HARM REDUCTION STRATEGIES TARGETING MODES OF ADMINISTRATION

As crystal may be snorted, swallowed, smoked, injected ("slamming"), and "booty bumped" (rectal administration), there are potential harms associated with each of these modes of administration. Harm reduction strategies may assist the client in assessing the harms of each method and increase understanding of the risks of each. Most of the crystal currently available on the street is "ice," a stronger form that is in a smokeable form–whether or not it is actually smoked (Inaba and Cohen, 2004). However, crystal is also frequently injected, particularly among gay male body builders who may already be injecting steroids (testosterone) and growth hormone. Consequently, harm reduction strategies may include a therapist discussing safer injection strategies, advising clients to "use a sterile syringe every time you inject and avoid sharing needles with others" (Sorge and Kershnar, 1998).

Harm Reduction Strategies When Clients Are Tweaking

Tweaking, or crystal intoxication, may last 8-12 hours, depending on the dose and purity; however, some users continue to use for days at a time. Symptoms of tweaking include:

- Teeth grinding, which may ultimately cause dental problems
- Sleep deprivation
- Severe paranoia
- Hallucinations, particularly auditory ones
- Perseveration
- Dissociaive trance states
- "Meth bugs" (paresthesias often described as bugs crawling under one's skin)
- Increased activity/performing repetitive acts
- Sexual dysfunction: either erectile dysfunction (colloquially known as "crystal dick") where the penis is semi-erect but shrunken; or impotence, the inability to achieve orgasm, or both.

This latter side effect of tweaking is worthy of particular, clinical attention. Given that users frequently say they use crystal because it facilitates sexual arousal and sexual activity, reminding them that crystal intoxication often interferes significantly with sexual performance provides an opportunity to explore costs and benefits of the drug–always with the goal of assisting the client in changing behavior. As crystal is widely known among tweakers to cause sexual dysfunction, users may combine crystal with sexual performance enhancing pharmaceuticals, such as Viagra (sildenafil) or Cialis (tadalafil). Among tweakers, the combination of crystal and Viagra is known as "trail mix."

Crystal use has been associated with HIV infection (Urbina and Jones, 2004; New York City Department of Health and Mental Hygiene, 2004). There are anecdotal reports that because of "crystal dick," sexually insertive gay and bisexual men ("tops") may change sexual roles and "bottom," which may increase their risk of acquiring HIV if having unprotected sex. Alternatively, gay and bisexual men who typically were "bottoms" may use sexual performance enhancing pharmaceuticals and function as "tops." In both cases, HIV-infected men engaging in unprotected anal sex (receptive or insertive) may place their uninfected sexual partners at risk. Crystal also may lead to behavior/identity discordance, in which males who identify as heterosexual may engage in sexual behaviors with other men while tweaking (MSM).

Clinicians need to assess all of the above behaviors with their clients in a non-judgmental manner if they are to intervene effectively regarding behavior change. As crystal impairs abstract cognitive functions, perceptions of risks and consequences, such as engaging in unprotected sex while tweaking, are frequently absent (Kingston and Conrad, 2004). It has been suggested in the literature that because of these deficits, accommodations be made if clinicians encounter clients who are tweaking (Kingston and Conrad, 2004). However, based upon the anecdotal experiences of staff at syringe exchange programs who encounter clients who tweak, clients may still be able to retain information, take free condoms, and verbalize intentions to engage in behavior change. Binge reduction strategies are important for clinicians to utilize as well because using crystal over several days may increase the likelihood of psychotic episodes (Semple, Patterson and Grant, 2003). A harm reduction goal might be to assist the client in using for one night, rather than non-stop for several days.

Health Concerns and Harm Reduction

Notable symptoms of withdrawal, or "crashing," from crystal include extreme exhaustion, sleep disorders, suicidal depression and increased anxiety. Given the profound nature of crystal withdrawal, "crash avoidance," in which users continue using, despite physical and mental health symptoms, is common (Halkitis, Parsons, and Stirratt, 2001). When crashing, crystal users often use sleeping pills and benzodiazepines ("downs") or opiates to alleviate withdrawal.

The consequences of long-term crystal use may include addiction, sexual compulsivity, emphysema from smoking crystal, coronary problems, HIV and syphilis. Injectors of crystal are also at increased risk of becoming infected with Hepatitis C.

Harm reduction strategies of intervention can target physical health concerns that may be expressed by the client or observed by the clinician, such as marked weight loss, dermatological problems, or depression. Clinicians can develop discrepancy in a non-judgmental manner by asking if health and mental health problems are worth the short-term expectations and challenging some of the likely distortions or defense mechanisms, such as minimization. Clinicians can also focus on HIV to motivate behavior change, even if this is not the presenting issue (McVinney, 2004).

Gay-Specific Harm Reduction Interventions

There is a compelling body of literature that argues for expanded access to drug treatment and specifically, treatment facilities for gay and bisexual men that are staffed by openly gay men (U.S. Department of Health and Human Services, 2001; Cabaj, 1996; Warn, 1997). Harm Reduction programs also need to be expanded and include gay specific programming (Task Force on Crystal Meth, Syphilis and HIV, 2004). Gay affirmative drug treatment programs are able to address the impact of homophobia and heterosexism, oppression, stigma management, intimacy and relationship issues (Neisen, 1997). Studies have found that when gay men seek treatment in a gay program, the outcomes are better (Cabaj, 1996).

Other diversity issues that may be addressed by clinicians include: (1) addressing co-occurring disorders such as sexual compulsivity; (2) developmental issues and the differences regarding crystal use among older versus younger gay men; (3) HIV status (the reasons for using crystal for HIV positive men may be different than for HIV negative men, or those with unknown status; (4) race and ethnicity; (5) socioeconomic status; and (6) MSM and bisexuality (McVinney, 2001). For crystal users who have become socially isolated and marginalized as a result of their drug use, assisting them in identifying other environments for socializing is enormously important and can reduce feelings of isolation. For these clients, a group modality may be indicated. This could include group psychotherapy, self-help groups like Crystal Meth Anonymous (CMA), and psychoeducational groups that focus on crystal meth.

Psychological Focus

Psychological problems associated with crystal use have been identified in the literature (Urbina and Jones, 2004) and may include: (1) mood disorders (notably major depression); (2) low self-esteem and low self-efficacy, especially following a binge or relapse; (3) anxiety disorders; (4) sleep disorders; (5) cognitive impairment; and (6) paranoia and psychosis. From a harm reduction perspective, these mental health concerns should be addressed without demanding that a client stop using crystal, but rather addressed by a clinician in a dual-focused manner (Kingston and Conrad, 2004).

Psychosocial Quality of Life Focus

There are numerous quality of life issues related to crystal use that can be addressed using a harm reduction perspective. Conceptualizing harm reduction as a form of health promotion that uses a strengths perspective, one asks clients if their current drug use is what they wanted from their lives and if this is how they envisioned their lives going. Such an approach may offer clients an opportunity to begin addressing their crystal use. Psychosocial issues include but are not limited to: (1) addiction and recovery (managing a chronic condition); (2) living with HIV infection; (3) lack of adherence to medications; (4) increased rates of STI's, notably syphilis; and (5) escalating associations with violence from drug dealing and dealers, involvement with hustlers and escorts, intimate partner violence, and gun violence (perhaps correlated with paranoia and aggression). All of these need to be assessed and can be addressed in a harm reduction framework.

CONCLUSIONS

Clinicians working with gay men using crystal meth would do well to embrace a harm reduction perspective that includes a continuum of strategies from safer use to abstinence. This article has defined harm reduction and described models of harm reduction interventions for crystal meth using gay men. Clinicians are encouraged to expand their knowledge about harm reduction. In addition, clinicians should become familiar with existing resources for treating crystal use (journals, books, internet), particularly those that advocate harm reduction.

REFERENCES

Bradley-Springer, L. (1996), Patient education for behavior change: Help from the transtheoretical and harm reduction models. *J. Association of Nurses in AIDS Care*, 7:23-40.

Brocato, J. & Wagner, E.F. (2003), Harm reduction: A social work practice model and social justice agenda. *Health & Social Work*, 28(2):117-125.

Cabaj, R. P. (1996), Substance abuse in gay men, lesbians, and bisexuals. In: *Textbook of Homosexuality and Mental Health*, eds. R.P. Cabaj & T.S. Stein. Washington, DC: American Psychiatric Press, pp. 783-800.

Des Jarlais, D.C. (1995), Harm reduction–a framework for incorporating science into drug policy. *American J. Public Health*, 85(1):10-13.

Freese, T.E., Miotto, K. & Rebeack, C.J. (2002), The effects and consequences of selected clubdrugs. *J. Substance Abuse Treatment,* 23:51-156.

Gay Men's Health Crisis (2004), *Crystal: What You Need to Know.* New York: Gay
Men's Health Crisis. http://www.gmhc.org/programs/crystal.html

Guss, J.R. (2000), Sex like you can't even imagine: "Crystal," crack, and gay men. *J.
Gay & Lesbian Psychotherapy,* 3(3/4): 105-122. Reprinted in *Addictions in the Gay
and Lesbian Community,* eds. J.R. Guss & J. Drescher. New York: The Haworth
Press, Inc., pp. 105-122.

Halkitis, P.N., Parsons, J.T. & Wilton, L. (2003), An exploratory study of contextual
and situational factors related to methamphetamine use among gay and bisexual
men in New York City. *J. Drug Issues,* 33(2):413-432.

Halkitis, P.N., Parsons, J.T. & Stirratt, M. (2001), A double epidemic: Crystal metham-
phetemine use and its relation to HIV prevention among gay men. *J. Homosexuality,* 41:17-35.

Harm Reduction Coalition (2005), Definition of harm reduction. Retrieved from http://
www.harmreduction.org.

Housenbold Seiger, B. (2003), Harm reduction: Is it for you? *J. Social Work Practice
in the Addictions,* 3(3):119-121.

Inaba, D.S. & Cohen, W.E., eds. (2004), *Uppers, Downers, All Arounders: Physical
and Mental Effects of Psychoactive Drugs.* 5th edition. Ashland, OR: CNS Publications.

Kingston, S. & Conrad, M. (2004), Harm reduction for methamphetamine users. *Focus. A Guide to AIDS Research & Counseling,* 19(1):5-6.

MacCoun, R.J. (1998), Toward a psychology of harm reduction. *American Psychologist,* 11:1199-1208.

McVinney, D. (2004), Motivational interviewing and psychotherapy. *Focus. A Guide
to AIDS Research & Counseling,* 19(7):5-6.

McVinney, L.D. (2001), Clinical issues with bisexuals. In: *A Provider's Introduction
to Substance Abuse Treatment for Lesbian, Gay, Bisexual, and Transgender Individuals.* Rockville, MD: U.S. Department of Health and Human Services, Center
for Substance Abuse Treatment.

Miller, W.R. & Rollnick, S., eds. (1991), *Motivational Interviewing: Preparing People
to Change Addictive Behavior.* New York: Guilford Press.

Miller, W.R. & Rollnick, S., eds. (2002), *Motivational Interviewing: Preparing People
for Change,* 2nd edition. New York: Guilford Press.

Neisen, J.H. (1997), An inpatient psychoeducational group model for gay men and les-
bians with alcohol and drug abuse problems. In: *Chemical Dependency Treatment:
Innovative Group Approaches,* ed. L.D. McVinney. Binghamton, NY: The Haworth
Press, Inc., pp. 37-51.

New York City Department of Health and Mental Hygiene (2004), Health bulletin:
Methamphetamine and HIV. *Health & Mental Hygiene News,* 3(3):unpaginated.

Owen, F. (2004), No man is a crystal meth user unto himself. *New York Times,* Section
9, pp. 1,10, August 29. http://www.nytimes.com/2004/08/29/fasion/29meth.html

Reback, C.J. (1997), *The Social Construction of a Gay Drug: Methamphetamine Use
Among Gay and Bisexual Males in Los Angeles.* Los Angeles: City of Los Angeles,
AIDS Coordinator's Office.

Reback, C.J., Larkins, S. & Shoptaw, S. (2004), Changes in the meaning of sexual risk behaviors among gay and bisexual male methamphetamine abusers before and after drug treatment. *AIDS & Behavior*, 8(1):87-98.

Roberts, L.J. & Marlatt, G.A. (1999), Harm reduction. In: *Sourcebook on Substance Abuse. Etiology, Epidemiology, Assessment, and Treatment*, eds. P.J. Ott, R.E. Tarter & R.T. Ammerman. Boston: Allyn and Bacon, pp. 389-398.

Semple, S.J., Patterson, T.L. & Grant, I. (2003), Binge use of methamphetamine among HIV-positive men who have sex with men: Pilot data and HIV prevention implications. *AIDS Education & Prevention*, 15(2):133-147.

Shernoff, M. (2005), *Sex Without Condoms: Unprotected Sex, Gay Men, and Barebacking*. New York: Routledge.

Sorge, R. & Kershnar, S. (1998), *Getting Off Right. A Safety Manual for Injection Drug Users*. New York: Harm Reduction Coalition. http://www.harmreduction.org/gor.html.

Task Force on Crystal Meth, Syphilis and HIV (2004), *Confronting Crystal Methamphetamine Use in New York City. Public Policy Recommendations*. New York, Gay Men's Health Crisis, July.

Tatarsky, A. (2002), *Harm Reduction Psychotherapy: A New Treatment for Drug and Alcohol Problems*. Northvale, NJ: Jason Aronson Inc.

Urbina, A. & Jones, K. (2004). Crystal methamphetamine, its analogues, and HIV infection: Medical and psychiatric aspects of a new epidemic. *Clinical Infectious Diseases*, 38:890-894.

U.S. Department of Health and Human Services (2001), *A Provider's Introduction to Substance Abuse Treatment for Lesbian, Gay, Bisexual, and Transgender Individuals*. Rockville, MD: Center for Substance Abuse Treatment.

Van Wormer, K. & Davis, D.R. (2003), *Addiction Treatment: A Strengths Perspective*. Pacific Grove, CA: Brooks/Cole.

Warn, D.J. (1997), Recovery issues of substance-abusing gay men. In: *Gender & Addictions: Men and Women in Treatment*, eds. S.L.A. Straussner & E. Zelvin. Northvale, NJ: Jason Aronson Inc, pp. 385-410.

Zelvin, E. & Davis, D.R. (2001), Harm reduction and abstinence based recovery: A dialogue. *J. Social Work Practice in the Addictions*, 1(1):121-133.

Index

Page numbers followed by the letter "t" designate tables; numbers followed by the letter "f" designate figures.

BOOK ORDER FORM!

Order a copy of this book with this form or online at:
http://www.HaworthPress.com/store/product.asp?sku= 5816

Crystal Meth and Men Who Have Sex with Men
What Mental Health Care Professionals Need to Know

— in softbound at $17.95 ISBN-13: 978-0-7890-3248-5 / ISBN-10: 0-7890-3248-1.
— in hardbound at $34.95 ISBN-13: 978-0-7890-3247-8 / ISBN-10: 0-7890-3247-3.

COST OF BOOKS _____

POSTAGE & HANDLING _____
US: $4.00 for first book & $1.50
for each additional book
Outside US: $5.00 for first book
& $2.00 for each additional book.

SUBTOTAL _____

In Canada: add 7% GST. _____

STATE TAX _____
CA, IL, IN, MN, NJ, NY, OH, PA & SD residents
please add appropriate local sales tax.

FINAL TOTAL _____
If paying in Canadian funds, convert
using the current exchange rate,
UNESCO coupons welcome.

❏ **BILL ME LATER:**
Bill-me option is good on US/Canada/
Mexico orders only; not good to jobbers,
wholesalers, or subscription agencies.

❏ **Signature** _____

❏ **Payment Enclosed: $**_____

❏ **PLEASE CHARGE TO MY CREDIT CARD:**
❏ Visa ❏ MasterCard ❏ AmEx ❏ Discover
❏ Diner's Club ❏ Eurocard ❏ JCB

Account #_____

Exp Date_____

Signature_____
(Prices in US dollars and subject to change without notice.)

PLEASE PRINT ALL INFORMATION OR ATTACH YOUR BUSINESS CARD

Name

Address

City   State/Province   Zip/Postal Code

Country

Tel   Fax

E-Mail

May we use your e-mail address for confirmations and other types of information? ❏Yes ❏No We appreciate receiving
your e-mail address. Haworth would like to e-mail special discount offers to you, as a preferred customer.
We will never share, rent, or exchange your e-mail address. We regard such actions as an invasion of your privacy.

Order from your **local bookstore** or directly from
The Haworth Press, Inc. 10 Alice Street, Binghamton, New York 13904-1580 • USA
Call our toll-free number (1-800-429-6784) / Outside US/Canada: (607) 722-5857
Fax: 1-800-895-0582 / Outside US/Canada: (607) 771-0012
E-mail your order to us: orders@HaworthPress.com

For orders outside US and Canada, you may wish to order through your local
sales representative, distributor, or bookseller.
For information, see http://HaworthPress.com/distributors

(Discounts are available for individual orders in US and Canada only, not booksellers/distributors.)

Please photocopy this form for your personal use.
www.HaworthPress.com

BOF06